■Searching for **The** Diet, Americans spend $5 billion annually - and are still looking. The search turned into a "weight-loss campaign" a long time ago. Yet this means completely missing the point!!! The **Diet** should be a regimen that keeps or makes you healthy - and sheds the extra weight, if there is any.

■Did you know that obesity, overweight, premature aging, heart attacks, strokes, cancers, osteoporosis, diabetes (Type II), constipation, diverticulitis, appendicitis, cavities, hypertension, hypoglycemia, heartburn, and ulcers are virtually unknown in some areas of the world?

■Did you know that almost all of these diseases are self-inflicted and easily preventable?

■Did you know that we are bombarded daily with misconceptions about fitness and disease-prevention?

■Do you have any idea what you are "fed" when you eat or drink?

■No, we have not come up with anything "revolutionary". We "just" compiled here what we learned during our research and visits in 21 countries about the contributing factors to a long, healthy and happy life.

■Discover the life-style of those who have the highest average life span in the world. Follow the path of these centenarians; they offer you 4 billion years of expertise in healthy living.

There is no way to guarantee how much healthier and longer this guide will make you live, but your life would definitely be shorter without it!

LIVE 100 HAPPY YEARS !
YOUR *PERSONAL* HEALTH GUIDE

BASED ON THE WISDOM
OF THE
LONG-LIVING
PEOPLES
OF THE WORLD

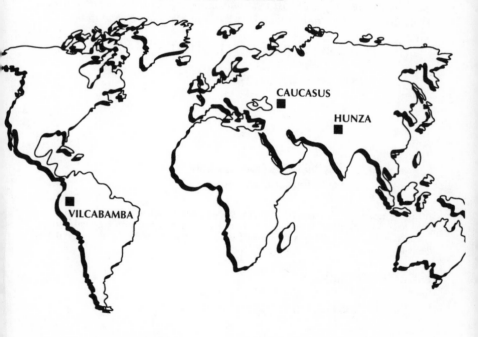

GLOBAL RESEARCH INSTITUTE

SANTA BARBARA, CALIFORNIA

NOTE

The information and recommendations in this health guide serve general educational purposes, and are not meant in any way to substitute for medical care or advice from qualified sources.

Global Research Institute strongly advises the reader to consult qualified medical doctors in case of any sign of ill health, or if the reader intends to apply any of the recommendations in this health guide. We do not assume responsibility or liability for any consequences of the failure of the reader to do so.

REQUEST

We would like to give the public the best, simplest and handiest health guide possible. Since there is always room for improvements, your comments (positive or negative) are most welcome. If you can contribute with any idea to the health of our children and the general public, please write to:

GLOBAL RESEARCH INSTITUTE
P.O.Box 50555
Santa Barbara, Ca. 93150

ISBN 0-9619630-1-8

Printed in the United States of America

CONTENTS

Preface..4

Introduction..6

The Life-Style of the Long-Living in Vilcabamba, Ecuador.......................10

The Life-Style of the Long-Living in the Caucasus.......................12

The Life-Style of the Long-Living in Hunza 20

Comparison..22

Substances that Make Up Our Body....................25

The Food We Eat - The Way We Live........................53

The "Avoid!" List..68

Only You Can Do It!..71

Now, What?..72

Make It a Habit!..77

Physical Activity..79

Stress..81

Children...82

This Is the Only Way to Do It!................................84

The "Smart Man's Diet"..85

Awareness Calendar..94

Bibliography..105

PREFACE

It is not our intention to sell or endorse any commercial product or to promote any specific "health improving" method. All the information compiled in this nutritional health guide is documented, and the sources are easily verifiable.

In the course of our research work on the subject, we were trying to be as careful as we possibly could to gather and rely on only relevant and unbiased information. This was undoubtedly a very hard task, considering the seemingly limitless sea of health related literature.

Despite our dedication and thorough commitment to giving the public the best health guide possible, we were both shocked and frustrated by the overabundance of medical and health books, magazines, brochures, and articles. In a library, for instance, you can walk between walls of books all related to health. Equally frustrating is their "thoroughness". If a book is about vitamin A or fish oil, a ton of information will be dumped on the reader, who will be left with the impression that a higher intake of these substances will solve all his problems.

Consider all the books, tapes and pills aimed at "controlling" appetite and weight. It is really incredible to see that in this gigantic weight control campaign, that costs consumers five billion dollars annually, nothing is said about the truth. The sad truth is that *we Americans have totally missed the point*. Most (but not all) of those "diets" really can make you slim - but not healthy! They offer the alternatives of staying on the "diet", which would shortly lead to self-destruction, or of going back to the original regimen which led to this sad situation in the first place. Many people are bouncing between the two "alternatives".

Understanding and utilizing other books dealing with wider aspects of health, require the knowledge of a medical doctor and the willpower of a world-class athlete. Ads, television commercials, friends, and fellow workers are bombarding us with advice as to what to eat or drink.

Who should we listen to? How can we find the right advice? Little can be questioned about the ability of science to determine the energy, vitamin, fiber or mineral content of any nutrition. However, as to how much of and how frequently these substances should be consumed, and their combined effects on the most sophisticated system in the Universe, the Human Body, these are questions nobody can answer. Even experts often contradict each other on these matters, and quite understandably, since the way billions and billions of cells are made up in our body and their interactions are truly mind-boggling.

At that point, we were even more convinced than before that a concise but still very simple, practical health guide should be given to everyone in this country for everyday use. We also wanted to provide *health advice that has credibility and is based on fact*. For advice of unshakeable credibility, where better to turn than to the facts of life displayed by long-living people in different parts of the world?

As you can see, it is not our intention to impress you with the thickness of our book. Here you will not find hard to understand medical terminology, "scientific" exercise programs, "how-to-lose-fifty-pounds-in-two-days-while-you-sleep" diets, or daily calorie charts (most of us have enough numbers to worry about). Despite the recipes, it is not meant to be a cookbook. Again, size, order, wording, printing, recipes - all were subjected to the basic idea of creating a down-to-earth health guide for everyday use.

We view the longevity of the people discussed in this guide as the *indisputable evidence for the life-prolonging, disease-preventing effects* of various substances and physical activities. We hope that both old and young users of this booklet will agree with us, and they will see our approach as a solid basis they can trust. In all likelihood, this will give them confidence and power in changing their life-style for the healthier.

INTRODUCTION

Take a few seconds and think of a chain that goes back in time; think of your parents and their parents and their parents... All those people are related to you. You are the way you are because you inherited everything from them; not only the color of your hair, but the ability to walk, to think, to talk, to see, to hear, to feel, and to fight diseases... But go back more than just three generations, go back 10, 200, 500 or 1000 generations, and now we are back about 40-50,000 years ago. At any given time there was a couple related to you. To name your relationship to them, who knows how many times the word "grand" should be put in front of "parent". They were hunting; they were hunted; they were cold, hungry, sick, scared... day after day, night after night. They saw others being butchered and eaten up by other creatures, and yet others drowning, freezing to death, or dying of disease. But these two survived till they produced offsprings, because they were lucky, and mainly because their predecessors (who are directly related to you also) had to go through the same hardship.

This chain could be followed all the way back to hundreds of millions of years for every one of us, back to the day when Nature or God made two atoms couple up and attract more atoms to create a cell. That particular cell is your relative. Even today, thousands of millions of years later, we start from one cell. Every baby in the mother's womb, starting from a cell, in nine months goes through all the phases that our forebears went through. The difference is that each phase of evolution lasted tens or hundreds of millions of years. It might sound like a pointless story, but it is not.

Think about how much hardship your forebears had to go through and suffer cold, hunger, and disease. Think of all the billions of nights and days of misery. But your ancestors were tough, tougher than anybody else. *Be proud of them*!

Now, here you are, their final product. You inherited everything from them; your ability to be a Human Being, the ability to love others, to enjoy a long, happy life. All the millions of your ancestors would be happy to see you have this chance. They suffered for you, but none of them had the chance you have.

We ought to express our appreciation and gratitude to our forebears for the hardship they endured for us, for all the abilities, toughness and the immune system they created for us during their endless sufferings.

Without a doubt, our body is strong. What an amazing system! It can last 40, 50, 60, sometimes even 70 years, despite all our efforts to destroy it through terrible eating and drinking habits, smoking, alcohol, smog, chemicals, stress, lack of physical activity, and drugs. Our body was not made to handle all this. Can you imagine how well it would do if we took care of it? Our forebears "put in a few working hours" to make it last 100 years. It does have the potential to last up to 100 years.

What do we do with our most precious heritage? *In this country, close to one million people die of heart attacks or other blood vessel diseases annually*, which means one of the highest mortality rates in this respect in the world. *The cancer toll is close to half a million deaths a year*. Of course, there are millions of other cases when the persons do not die but suffer long-term ill-effects. *The rate of women dying from heart diseases is the highest in the U.S.*

Blood vessel diseases seem to be reaching younger and younger people, people in their forties, even thirties. This fast-paced life-style accelerates biological processes so much that people in their thirties, forties and fifties succumb to diseases normally associated with older age (eighty, ninety). The total financial cost of the civilization diseases is estimated to be around 100 billion dollars annually in the U.S.

Contrary to popular belief, between fifty to ninety percent of these tragedies are caused by external factors, and most of them can be prevented. For example, with a minor switch in the diet, diabetes can be prevented or even cured in most cases, but still the life of five to six million people in the U.S. is shortened by this disease.

Despite the proximity of hospitals and the availability of the most sophisticated medical technology, in this country people are dying needlessly even while you are reading this sentence. We tend to consider these premature deaths something unavoidable.

Undoubtedly, Nature gives us approximately one hundred years to live. What do we do with our once-and-only life? Destroy it. How? Through ignorance. When someone says, "I don't care, everybody has to die of something, and I would rather enjoy life in the meantime," it doesn't mean that he doesn't care. It means he does not know how to care. Life can be just as full and enjoyable when one knows how to care for his health, how to lead a little bit more sensible life-style. The tragedies mentioned do not happen only to others; it is coming; it will happen to you and every one of us if we do not learn how to care for ourselves.

Your health is your future, your healthy body and mind will be the subject and source of joy for a long time to come. Every year, millions of people suddenly have to face the shocking reality: their life will end very soon. It happens to all of us earlier or later in our life. The most alarming thing about it is the new appearance of the "civilization diseases": *blood vessel diseases, cancers and diabetes cut the life of younger and younger people in half in increasing numbers despite the advancement of civilization.*

You might be one of the lucky ones who do not have health problems yet. Still, think about the terrible feeling when the never-expected tragedy is here, and you have to "revise" your plans for the future. There are no more plans; there are no more things to look forward to; you have to leave your parents, friends and everything you love behind. Undescribable misery! Real people make up the statistics. This will happen to you, too, if you do not know how to care for your health.

Why does a 47-year-old, seemingly healthy, strong person have to die of cancer, or heart attack? And not only one, but millions of them. It does not have to be that way. Most of us devote more attention to our cars than to our health. That is why we leave behind shiny cars and everything else we worked so hard for in our short(ened) life.

Be more aware of your responsibility for your health, for your life! Nobody else will do it for you. Try to copy the life-style of the long-living people as much as possible.

Certainly one may ask, "what can we have in common with these people hidden in distant corners of the earth, living in the Stone Age by our standards?" Undoubtedly, there are numerous differences, but the very remoteness, their "isolatedness" might have preserved principal truths of health that the "civilized man" easily forgets.

The longevity of the folks we have studied is ample proof that they indeed have preserved the way of life which causes or at least contributes to good health and long life. We trust that many will agree with us that there could be no more trustworthy "authority" than these long-living peoples in deciding which is the healthiest life-style and diet.

Listen to them attentively!

THE LIFE-STYLE OF THE LONG-LIVING IN VILCABAMBA, ECUADOR

In the rugged mountainous terrain of southern Ecuador, there is a small pocket of people with an extremely high ratio of elderly. They live in a small village called Vilcabamba at an elevation of about 4500 feet, surrounded by the high mountains of the Andes.

The 1971 census found 9 persons over 100 years of age out of a population of 819. From baptismal records, their age was determined with reasonable accuracy. The U.S. rate is 3 out of 100,000. Ecuadorian doctors reported 1 person of 65 or older out of every 6 - double the number in the U.S.

These people have never had medical services available to prolong their life. Medical experts have studied them, especially those who had lived over 100 years. With very few exceptions, *no evidences of blood vessel disease or other serious health problems were found among these centenarians.* Some of them suffer heart attacks, but show no symptoms, they carry on with their life as if nothing had happened. Very few of them have had broken bones ever, and even the oldest ones are leading a normal life, perfectly able to take care of themselves.

According to blood tests, the people in this village are of mixed race, they have the blood of Europeans and American Indians in their veins. While there is no doubt that genetic diversity is likely to produce more resistant members in any species, most of us in almost any part of the world have this "advantage". Good mixture of genes, obviously, cannot explain their longevity.

Their diet is very "poor" by our standards in variety, quantity, and quality. They eat whatever is found around the house: corn, beans, barley, wheat, fruits, nuts, wild berries, vegetables (carrots, turnips, lettuce, sweet potatoes, yucca, etc.). Meat, milk, cheese and eggs are scarce, consumed seldom and in very small quantities. The latter are what people in the affluent societies consider indispensable ingredients of a "well-balanced, nutritious" meal (three times a day if possible), since they are the sources of "vital" animal proteins.

Instead, these centenarians *rely on mainly beans, corn, fruits and vegetables and live happily up to 100 years and even longer.*

Their average energy intake is about 1200 calories a day, as opposed to over 3000 calories in the U.S. We eat about three times as much protein, about ten times as much fat, altogether about three times as much calories as they do - and work physically about three times less than they do. It is no wonder there is not one overweight among the long-living, and about half of our population are considered overweight.

Drinking alcoholic beverages and smoking are not common at all, practiced by only a few with moderation. Simple lard is used for cooking, but there is never enough around for deep-frying.

One can summarize the regimen of these centenarians as a *near-vegetarian* diet. Animal supplied foods, even milk, are considered delicacies due to their scarcity. Beans, corn, fruits, potatoes and vegetables are dominant. They make their own whole-wheat bread. Their meals are not "well-balanced" even in the limited sense: they do not have all the food groups in the same meal, not even every day, as is suggested by most of our dieticians. Modest meals three to four times a day is the normal. They can be described as "undernourished".

The other chief characteristic of their life-style is their astonishing agility. *Not running, not jogging, but walking is what they are doing all day, every day.* Working around the house, walking up and down to the corn fields, working there all day, walking home again, going to bed early - this is their typical daily activity. Walking long distances, uphill or downhill, is part of their daily life. Even people over 100 years old keep busy, keep walking and working all day long. They are able to take care of themselves till their last days.

THE LIFE-STYLE OF THE LONG-LIVING IN THE CAUCASUS

The Caucasus is a high mountain range between Europe and Asia, connecting the Black and the Caspian Seas. The area is part of the Soviet Union. In about a dozen so-called autonomous republics and regions live over two hundred ethnic groups. The population of the groups varies from a few thousand to several million (Georgia, Armenia, Azerbaijan).

Many tribes, nations, and armies moved through this great gate during human history, mixing with each other and the local people; some of them settled permanently. Mongols, Arabs, Greeks, Romans, Jews, Russians, and who knows how many more are represented here. These people definitely have the advantage genetic diversity offers.

The truly outstanding feature of these folks, besides their cheerfulness and hospitality, is the high number of long-living among them. *The largest concentration of centenarians in the world* is found in the low-lying valleys, in the foothills, and the high mountains of the Caucasus. Thirty to forty, in some areas fifty to one hundred centenarians per every 100,000 people have been reported in the region, which is ten to thirty times the number we can count in the U.S. (3 per 100,000). This clearly shows that the natural limit of life for an average human being is around one hundred years.

Almost without exception, despite being a century old (or some even older), they are more active in everyday life, more self-reliant, and have better mental attitude than many people in their sixties or seventies in other countries. They move along all day, tending the garden, the poultry, the household, herding the sheep. They spend most of their time outdoors, even sleep outside, if the weather permits. Taking a nap after lunch is fairly common, despite the fact that constant physical activity makes them sleep well and long at night (seven to ten hours). A slow-paced, unhurried, orderly life-style it is.

It should be noted that the long-living are distributed unevenly in this diverse region. The percentage of elderly in the foothills is several times higher than in the valleys and plains; in the mountains (1000-4500 feet), it is even higher than in the foothills.

There seems to be a close inverse correlation between the incidences of blood vessel diseases and the elevation at which the studied people live. The directly contributing factor is not the elevation itself, but the life-style different groups are forced to adapt to. The higher we go, the farther we get from "civilization", and the more people seem to have succeeded in preserving the traditional way of life. It means constant physical work, and *a great deal of climbing and walking*, as part of the daily life. No, they are not moving mountains or digging tunnels through solid rock, but simply have to walk if they want to get somewhere, have to weed the garden if they want to make a living.

The diet pattern shows more of a horizontal rather than a vertical variation.

Let us start with our arch-enemies: meat and fat. Yes, these folks invariably like to include meat in their diet. Among the highest mountains of Azerbaijan, mutton fried with fat is a favorite; beef and chicken are consumed, also. Foods rich in (animal) fat do not seem to be an obstacle in their way to older ages. They show an incredible longevity ratio: over 500 centenarians per 100,000 in some places. Smoking is used as a way to preserve meat for seasons when it is more scarce. No edible part of an animal is wasted; the organs are turned into spicy, delicious sausages; bones produce tasty soups and sauces.

In eastern Georgia, melted sheep fat is preferred over vegetable fat; whereas, the western part of the republic uses mainly walnut as shortening. The average total calorie intake is nearly equal (1800-2000 calories a day), but the easterners consume about twice as much meat, wheat products, and sugar as the westerners. On the other hand, the western part eats mainly honey for sweets, boiled meat instead of fried, and twice as much milk products. The average life span is noticably higher in the western part.

Boiling meat is provenly more beneficial, as this method of preparation makes meat easier to digest. For older persons whose enzyme activity in the glands has decreased, it is of great importance. It is interesting that folks in western Georgia and Azerbaijan avoid using the broths produced as they boil meat, wasting a great deal of minerals and other substances. Obviously, they make up for it by consuming alternative sources, like milk products, vegetables, fruits - and, of course, they eat the meat they cook.

Aside from the rest of their diet, *there is an extremely important common factor in their meat eating habits: they do not eat much*.

It is amusing how some researchers are misled by the local custom of slaughtering an animal at the arrival of a respected guest. A sheep or perhaps just a chicken is sacrificed not to the honor of the guest or because these folks "prefer everything fresh". They do it out of necessity; they can afford to eat meat only on rare occasions, which can be a holiday or any special event like the birth of a child - or even a visit by a guest. Letting the animal live until the time comes is a way to preserve the scarce meat.

Of course, in the last few decades the frequency of meat consumption has reached the once-a-week level. That is where the Eastern European countries were 20-30 years ago, and then meat became more plentiful there. Now, after eating lots of meat for 20-30 years, Nature's "grace period" expiring, they are doing what their economy could not do: they are catching up with the West - in dying of civilization diseases.

The average calorie intake in the Caucasus (about 1800-2000 a day) is slightly higher than in Vilcabamba (1200-1400) but still about one third less then the U.S. average. Most importantly, only 5-20% of these calories come from animal fat, as opposed to 50-80% in the U.S.

Now, let us take a look at the part of their eating habits that perhaps has the most to do with their longevity. Actually, there are numerous common factors that clearly expand their life span.

Processed foods were unheard-of until very recent times. Nearly all the vegetables and fruits are eaten fresh or after slight alteration. Truly remarkable is the large amount of fermented dairy products consumed every day: sour milk and yogurt-like variations, light cheeses, skim whey, cottage cheese. These are rich sources of important vitamins, minerals and proteins. Yogurt is frequently diluted and drunk with water, or mixed with garlic and eaten with other dishes.

They use cow, sheep or goat milk - but seldom without fermentation. This process breaks down the hard-to-digest substances in the fresh milk. After this change (as yogurt or kefir, for example), milk seems to play a highly beneficial role in helping digestion, making bones stronger by its high calcium content, providing easy-to-digest proteins and vital mineral salts. Perhaps most importantly, it reduces blood cholesterol levels.

This last merit of fermented milk products could be an explanation for the low blood cholesterol levels and high resistance to heart disease observed among the Masai tribesmen in East Africa. Of course, walking after their cattle 10 to 20 miles a day should also contribute to the virtual absence of heart disease among them. (*U.S. laboratory tests have proven the ability of yogurt to lower the level of cholesterol in the blood stream of humans*).

As a result of their nomadic way of life, the tribesmen do not cultivate much land, and that is where the people of the Caucasus have the winning edge: they get more fruits and vegetables. Looking back to Vilcabamba, one can easily detect the similarity: those centenarians have had no access to plenty of milk and meat products, sustain themselves mainly on plant supplied foods, and still live 100 (or even more) happy years.

In the light of all this, it is obvious: fruits and vegetables play a role of vital importance in our life.

The most important feature of the Caucasian diet is definitely the dominance of unprocessed, natural foods of plant origin. The wide category of "plant origin" is profoundly justifiable, since it comprises an incredible variety of vegetables, fruits, berries, herbs, spices, nuts, grains, dry legumes, and every conceivable edible plant part.

It ought to be emphasized that these people are far from being vegetarian, although, for practical and religious reasons, different groups prefer or abstain from eating certain animals. Moslems and the Mountain Jews are prohibited by their religions from keeping or eating pigs. Others include pork in their diet. Beef is generally accepted, but cattle are more demanding as to the quality of the grazing land. Poultry is kept in almost every household. But, the uncontested favorite is mutton, understandably, since sheep is most suitable for that climate and terrain.

We should keep in mind, though, that the daily regimen of an average person consists predominantly of vegetables. They cook vegetables with legumes, dairy products, or meat (occasionally), but large portions are eaten in the form of different salads several times a day - even in the morning. Lettuce, tomato, green beans and peas, sorrel, garlic, cucumber, peppers, celery, cabbage, squash, potato, radishes, eggplant, pumpkin, carrot, parsley, and beets are among those used.

Vegetables are easy to cultivate; a small plot can provide even a large family with all they need for a whole year. If one produced more, the surplus can be sold on the market to those who for some reason have to buy at least part of their supplies; like shepherds who are herding their sheep up in the mountains most of the year.

With the exception of the low-lying valleys, the production is seasonal, and from this arises the necessity to preserve as much as possible for winter and early spring. It is the responsibility of the female members of the family to conserve vegetables, fruits, wild berries and herbs as they ripen one after the other. Naturally, the children are great help in gathering and preparation. These activities require a great deal of attention, planning and sometimes strenuous, physical work, but it is a natural part of the yearly life-cycle as is getting out of bed every morning.

Some vegetables are pickled or dried; some are simply put in dark places of even temperature. People do not necessarily have all the kinds of vegetables readily available all the time despite their effort and planning during the growing season. When they run out of one kind, more of others are used. One thing is certain: they always want to make sure that they will not run out of everything before the next season arrives. All this naturally applies to fruits as well.

Fruit trees need more space, and it may be 3 to 5 years before they start bringing fruit. It is general practice to utilize the space by growing vegetables, melons and pumpkins among the trees. Plums, apricots, apples, peaches, cherry, tart cherry, figs, pomegranates, oranges, lemons, and grapes are the most popular whether raw or some of them cooked.

No day goes by without eating large amounts of fruits and vegetables, which are rich sources of energy, minerals, vitamins, fiber and liquid.

With meat being only a delicacy on weekends, holidays and special events, grains, legumes and potato (along with dairy products) are the main sources of proteins, energy, additional vitamins, minerals and fiber.

Legumes (a wide variety of beans, peas, and lentils) are very popular all over the world, as they need no special care, and large quantities can be produced on even a small acreage. The Caucasus is no exception. When asked, many centenarians attribute their longevity to eating these "poor man's foods".

One cannot emphasize enough the importance of legumes in feeding humans and animals. In their ripened, dry form, they contain more protein than any other plant food, almost as much as meats have. *The carbohydrates in legumes give you a bit more calories than lean meat, but unlike meat, not all those calories are absorbable. Your body receives from legumes ten times more calcium, four times more potassium, three times more phosphorus and iron, and more vitamins than from meat - and almost no fat or cholesterol!* Meats contain no dietary fiber at all.

Eating legumes regularly, drastically improves the condition of people suffering from diabetes Type II (about 90 % of all diabetics !), diverticulosis or diverticulitis, regulates blood sugar levels, lowers blood cholesterol levels (while eating animal fat has a raising effect).

Legumes surpass almost any other type of food in fiber content, a dietary component whose "activities" are not fully understood by modern science, but it is a "sure suspect" in preventing cancer - just to mention one of its numerous merits.

A few amino acids are missing from legumes, and iron is not easily absorbed from them. Adding some whole-grain and dairy products to the menu takes care of the first problem, eating fruits and vegetables solves the second.

And what a "surprising coincidence": this is exactly what the people in the Caucasus are doing. For centuries, they have met their dietary requirements superbly through wisely combining the available foodstuffs. The traditionally scarce meat supply did not prevent them from reaching unusually high ages; on the contrary, it seems to have prolonged their life.

Mixing rice with meals made with dry legumes, adding dairy products or vegetables (sometimes meat), or just simply eating whole-grain bread with them are the ways all the long-living people combine these complementary nutrients.

We have to mention here that sending rice or other grains through a modern mill produces kernels almost completely stripped of their most valuable components: vitamins, minerals, essential fatty acids, and fiber. White flour made from stripped grains contain almost nothing else but fattening starches. On the other hand, the traditional milling process produces flours that have all the merits of the original grain.

Since refined grain products were not available until recently, these folks have been nourished by whole-grains all their life. Wheat, barley, rice, rye, oat, millet, and corn are grown in the area. It is customary there to make six-grain bread. Potato is also heavily cultivated and stored for winter and spring in large quantities.

A wide variety of dried and toasted seeds and nuts are eaten all year round. They are crushed or grated for seasoning or shortening. Walnut is used for cooking instead of animal fat in Abkhasia and western Georgia. Small as they are, the amount of vitamins, minerals, proteins and unsaturated fats that seeds and nuts have to offer is significant, especially in winter and early spring when other sources are scarce. Sunflower and pumpkin seeds, walnut, hazelnut, chestnut, almond, and pecan are ubiquitous.

Other seeds (coriander, anise, celery, poppy, etc.) are used in baking and cooking, together with numerous other popular food additives such as some vegetables, herbs, and spices.

These folks are ingenious in growing, gathering and utilizing spices and herbs. Wild-growing herbs are more commonly found and used by the people in the grazing lands and wooded areas up in the higher mountains. Imported spices are popular, as well, but with great care and devotion, many more are grown or picked in the wild locally.

Salt (with moderation), garlic (in almost everything), red peppers (hot and mild), black pepper, caraway seed, celery, parsley (roots and leaves), mint, nettle, chives, burdock, leek, sorrel, savory, cress compose a partial list. Most of them are surprisingly rich in vitamins and minerals, making the meals not only tastier but healthier as well. As a matter of fact, some of them are credited with medical properties. Garlic, for instance, has been used for centuries to cure several diseases; even modern medical science considers it a preventive medicine for the blood and digestive systems.

It is customary to drink teas brewed from the flowers of linden, strawberry, hawthorne, or rose hips.

These people have sweet tooth just like the rest of us, but for sweet fruits and berries, or natural honey - instead of ice cream or candies. They eat large quantities of grapes; it is not unusual for a person to eat 100 pounds of grape in a season.

The sugar in these "sweets" is different from our refined white crystals; the grape sugar (glucose) in fruits is transformed by the body into energy at a slower rate; whereas, the refined sugar is pure energy, carries no liquid, fiber or anything else but a rush of energy, destabilizing the blood sugar level. If the sweet calories are clad in their natural clothes, they can be beneficial.

Drinking the right drink in the right quantity at the right time is just as important as eating. In this respect the long-living have an easier "task" than we do: they are not exposed to the temptation of dozens of different kinds of sodas, juices and alcoholic beverages. Most of them drink only water, some mix it with yogurt or sour milk. Most men drink wine with moderation. Moslems prefer strong teas. Drunkenness is a shame, and the fear of being ashamed is more forceful than the law. A small amount of clear wine (about 2 glasses a day) is considered beneficial for digestion, but women and moslems, who do not drink at all, live just as long and are just as happy.

The majority of the centenarians have never smoked; the ones who did, quit when they were still "young", 50-70 years old.

Most of them have good teeth for most of their life. They eat regularly 3 to 4 times a day, and it is their custom to never eat to satiety. Sure enough, you can never see an overweight person among the old people.

THE LIFE-STYLE OF THE LONG-LIVING IN HUNZA

In northeastern Pakistan, where the Hindu Kush mountains meat the Himalayas, there is a small group of people who have gained world fame with their longevity and peculiar diet.

Nobody knows how long they have been living in this area called Hunza; their past is a mystery just like their language. They are not related to the neighboring tribes.

They must have settled there a long time ago, for Aryan tribes with light colored skin like theirs moved through the almost impassable area thousands of years ago. So, here we have individuals with relatively pure blood, without the "winning edge" of mixed races - and still they live to be 100 and even more.

British doctors started studying them even back in the thirties to reveal the "secret" of their longevity.

The steep mountains there are not suitable for herding many animals, so they raise goats and some sheep, but the source of their livelihood is agriculture. In the narrow valleys and the terraced hillsides every stretch of land is utilized. The people spend most of their time outdoors cultivating their plots or tending their animals.

Wheat, barley and millet are the primary crops. Their bread is always made with whole-grain flour. A variety of vegetables (carrot, turnip, parsley, etc.) are grown here, and eaten every day, and, of course, the indispensable legumes: beans, peas and lentils (green and dry).

The most intriguing part of their menu is the exceptionally high percentage of fruits (fresh or dried) in their regimen. Among the many kinds, *apricot* is the most popular. These folks not only survive on a diet that consists of bread, fermented milk, and apricot, but are able to work long hours in the fields, to walk miles up and down the steep hillsides every day - even when they are very old.

The work on the fields starts with an empty stomach; after 2-3 hours, the breakfast consists of: whole-grain bread, cottage cheese, and apricot (fresh or dried kneaded with water). The same routine is followed at lunch and sometimes even at dinner.

When in the season, fresh vegetables complement this lopsided regimen. Vegetables are slightly cooked in little water, and they always utilize the cooking water in some form.

They are experts at preserving fruits, especially the famous apricot, for winter and spring.

On the average, *they eat meat once every ten days*, so most of the time fermented dairy products supply the animal proteins. Very few chickens are kept, so practically no eggs are available.

No rice, tea, or refined sugar are consumed by these centenarians. Many (mostly children) show signs of undernourishment, especially in the spring before the next harvest arrives. They do not smoke, drink only water, milk and wine (with moderation).

The same British doctors conducted a very intriguiging experiment. Rats were fed a diet very similar to that of the long-living in Hunza. It included unboiled whole milk, sprouted *legumes*, fresh raw cabbage, carrot, *whole-wheat* bread with some fresh butter, and plenty of water every day; once a week the animals received a small amount of meat with some bones. After 27 months (the equivalent of about 55 years of age at man) the animals were perfectly healthy.

A control group of rats lived on *white (refined) rice*, legumes, vegetables, condiments, and just a little bit of milk - the diet of the poor people of Bengal and Madras states in India. These animals started showing signs of several diseases almost from the beginning: cancers, crooked spines, bad teeth, ulcers and so forth.

The third group which ate the typical English diet had even less luck. *White bread, sweetened tea, jams, canned meat*, boiled vegetables not only caused a wide variety of diseases in different parts of their body, but many showed symptoms of neurasthenia, nervousness and even cannibalism.

It does matter what you eat!

COMPARISON

We have studied the main characteristics of three groups of people who enjoy the greatest longevity on earth. There should be a reason why they do and others do not live up to 100 years in large numbers. Let us try to determine the common factor (or factors) that would lead us to understand this phenomenon of ultimate interest to all of us.

Since the groups live hundreds and even thousands of miles apart, it is highly unlikely that some unexplained element of the earth's crust, or perhaps the soil give them a "helping hand".

Although most of the longevious individuals are found in mountainous areas, thousands of them live close to sea level (near the Black Sea and the low-lying valleys of the Caucasus); so topography cannot explain it either. Most of their mountain settlements are at elevations not higher than 4500 feet. There is nothing special about it since millions of ordinary people live at the same level in other parts of the world.

The climate at Vilcabamba and the Black Sea is evenly mild, the mountains of the Caucasus and the Himalayas see snow every winter. During the winter, for instance, the people of Hunza spend their days in their huts half full with smoke, sitting around the open fire waiting for the spring sunshine.

Plains, mountains, summers, winters, clean air, smoky air, and sunshine are not limited to these areas, so none of these environmental factors seems to link all three groups together as the major and exlusive common contributor to their longevity.

Genetically they are not related to each other; most of them are mixtures of distant races. The exception is the people of Hunza who are considered a relatively pure race.

Obviously, the "secret linkage" lies in the individuals themselves, in the way they do things in their everyday life. And what do we do in our everyday life? Eat, drink, work, sleep.

What is common in their eating habits? First of all, *they do not eat too much, never to satiety,* just simply want to chase away the feeling of

hunger... *They are not vegetarians, but consume meat only occasionally.*
The exception could be some groups in the Caucasus with lots of animals,
who get more meat and animal fat, but the consumption of other foods
seems to offset the possible negative effects.

Dairy products are also important part of the diet - except in Vilcabamba.

*We can witness an ideal combination of foodstuffs: large amounts of
legumes accompanied with whole-grain products (unrefined rice, wheat,
maize or millet with beans, peas or lentils). This combination ensures a
steady supply of fiber, energy, vitamins and minerals, but most importantly,
all the amino acids needed by the body to build up the vital proteins.*

*All three groups eat a wide variety of foods, but fruits, vegetables, dry
legumes and whole-grains are clearly dominant.*

Processed foods are practically unknown among them. Fruit and
vegetable preservation is as natural as can be.

Lesson to be learned: eat little; eat mainly vegetables fruits, grains
and fermented dairy products, as little meat as possible; do not eat
processed (refined) food.

Drinking clear water is another link among them. It has been
proven by the peoples of the Caucasus and Hunza that drinking little
wine, tea, or teas brewed from certain wild berries cannot hurt, and even
can be beneficial.

Lesson to be learned: drink lots of water as clear as you can get;
eat fruits when no healthy drinks are available; 1 or 2 glasses of wine or
tea cannot hurt.

Very few of the long-living ever smoked; the ones who did, stopped
in time.

Lesson to be learned: quit! (Thirty million of us already did.)

These folks live a slow-paced, low-key life. Going to bed early, and sleeping 7-8 hours (even into old age) must also contribute to their vigorous health.

Lesson to be learned: do not neglect resting (but do not overdo it either).

Besides their diet, undoubtedly, the other chief reason for reaching such old ages in good health is their physical activities. Most of them have not run even a mile in the last 90 years of their life; on the other hand, they are are not sitting around idle hour after hour like most of us. Slow rhythmical movements (walking, gardening, housework) give them endurance and resilience - without big muscles.

Lessons to be learned: put your body to work so it will last, but do not overdo exercise (athletes do not live long).

SUBSTANCES THAT MAKE UP OUR BODY

Chances are that you are already familiar with at least the most important substances that make up our body. We still see it necessary to go through them one by one to ensure a clearer understanding of the ideas we are trying to get across to you in this health guide.

In compliance with our original approach, no recommended ounces, grams, and calories or recommended daily vitamin and mineral allowances are mentioned here, for it would confuse the issue of the *natural approach to genuine health, which our guide is meant to be.*

Even after thousands of experiments and epidemiological studies all over the world, scientists cannot agree as to the exact amounts of vitamins, minerals, hydrocarbons, fats, cholesterol, and proteins our bodies need. Even though experts do know that many substances are harmful, and many others are extremely important for the body, *"deficient" and "excessive" are still poorly defined terms even in scientific circles. There is a fair amount of confusion, to say the least.*

This confusion is reflected in the decisions of government officials "recommending" certain amounts of vitamins and minerals, or approving the use of thousands of chemicals in producing, processing and packaging foods and drinks. A shockingly high percentage of the applied chemicals have been proved to be cancer-causing in "larger doses". The bigger problem is that no one knows what "larger doses" means! Where does it start for the elderly, for the young, for the overweight, for the slim, for a baby, for the pregnant, for a fetus? No one knows.

One might say that everybody is eating and drinking the same foods and drinks, and there are still older people among us. That is true, but most of these chemicals have been introduced in the last few decades, and new ones are invented and applied at an accelerating rate.

All this applies not only to artificial preservatives or herbicides but to vitamin and mineral supplements and all the new fancy "formulas". **There is no safe chemical!**

There is one thing scientists can agree on: the best and the safest way to provide the body with all the vital substances is through eating natural food. Yes, let your body choose the kinds and quantities it needs. No one can beat 4 billion years of experience! Trust this experience, not the siren voice of the advertisements.

Now, let us see what our body has to have and what it has to cope with.

Proteins

Proteins are the building blocks of the body: nails, hair, skin, body organs and muscles are made of them. They are the "raw material" in "manufacturing" hormones and enzymes, and antibodies for the immune system.

Obviously, there is a need for a continuous supply to replace those that have worn out. Amino acids are the components that proteins are made of; their number and their particular arrangement will determine the resulting protein. We know of dozens of different amino acids, but only 22 of them are believed to be necessary for humans. Of the 22, the human body can produce only 14; the remaining 8 should be provided by the food we eat. (Some think 9 should be provided by outside sources). Animal supplied foods - meat, milk, eggs - are rich in proteins that contain all the "essential" (that is: missing) 8 (or 9?) amino acids; that is why animal proteins are called "complete".

On the other hand, most plants have proteins that are lacking one or more of the "essential" amino acids. Different plants are missing different ones, so that combining certain plants will provide the body with all the amino acids it needs to build its proteins. Eating legumes together with whole-grain foods is a good example. Combining of different food groups makes it possible for hundreds of millions of people to live on strict vegetarian diet all over the world. (It should be noted here, that *some scientists believe potatoes have all the essential amino acids*.)

Consuming too much protein-rich animal supplied foods is not a wise short-cut. The next chapters will tell more about it.

Carbohydrates

Carbohydrates are made up by carbon, hydrogen and oxygen molecules. Both simple (refined sugar) and complex carbohydrates (complex sugars, starches) are rich energy sources. Fats and proteins can also supply the body with energy, but they are harder to digest, and their residues are hard on the kidneys. Plants are rich in carbodydrates.

Dietary fiber

Undigestible carbohydrates and carbohydrate-like components of food (cellulose, pectin, etc.) - called: dietary fiber - have no direct nutritional value, but play a very beneficial role in helping the body to function properly. (More about dietary fiber later.)

Fats

Fats are very important for the body. Without them, the fat-soluble vitamins (A, D, E, K) cannot be utilized - just to mention one of their many functions.

Being almost pure energy, fats carry more calories than even refined sugar or alcohol. The problem is that a small amount, a spoonful of vegetable oil or butter a day, would do the job. Excessive fat intake will easily lead to overweight. *Every extra pound will require an additional 2 miles of blood vessels*, so that 20-pound "spare tire" many of us are tugging along means a lot of unnecessary strain on the heart.

Fats are also linked to higher cholesterol levels in the blood stream, a condition strongly suspected of contributing to heart attacks and other blood vessel diseases.

There are saturated, polyunsaturated, and monounsaturated fats. Until recently, scientists believed that only the first type raises the cholesterol level, and the two other lower it. Nowdays, they think that only monounsaturated fats (olive oil and peanut oil, to name two) decrease it.

Excess fat intake (regardless of the kind) promotes cancer growth. The example of the long-living has shown that safe fat is little fat.

Vitamins

Vitamins are chemical compounds needed in very small amounts to assist the body in processing and utilizing nutrients. Get your vitamins in their natural form, simply because nobody knows exactly how they work, interact, and how much of them is needed. Think of the long-living: they are almost undernourished, but doing fine without any medication or supplements.

The body is smarter than those who believe in excessive amounts of vitamins and/or minerals: it uses a certain amount and flushes out the rest. The problem is that fat-soluble vitamins and some minerals can accumulate in the system and cause serious ill-effects.

Vitamins are needed only in very small quantities. The root of the problem is that supplements are powerful concentrates, similarly to fats, refined sugar, or white flour which are concentrated energy. It is easy to take in too much of them, because they are readily available in the affluent societies.

Vitamins, minerals, fat, cholesterol, proteins, carbohydrates, etc. are best utilized when they are "wrapped up" in or accompanied by whole grains, fruits and vegetables, because the dietary fiber and the water in them prevent oversupply, and the body has a better control as to when, what and how much it will utilize. This is a simplified explanation, but it is essentially true. Our digestive system was molded in the last few million years by a near-vegetarian diet. This is how the human race survived, got strong and enabled itself to fight diseases, and this the way the long-living people do it.

In addition to their "normal" tasks, vitamins are indispensably help-ful in slowing down the aging process at molecular and cellular levels through preventing oxidation, so that cells can "breathe", and through deactivating free-radicals. *Free-radicals are very active, distorted molecules produced in the cells during normal functioning, but their number can be increased tremendously by outside effects*: smoking, alcohol, burned meals (meat, oils, etc.), pickled vegetables, smoked meat, and thousands of chemicals that get into our body through smog, polluted water, preservatives, hormones, tranquilizers, herbicides, pesticides, and other residues in our food, X-ray, etc. *Free-radicals are linked not only to wrinkled skin, but to cancers, hardened blood vessels and heart diseases, as well.*

Some vitamins seem to be more active than others in deactivating free-radicals and preventing oxidation in the cells. We still think that it would be a mistake to take large amounts of those vitamins (C and mainly E) in the form of supplements. The minimum danger we see is that it will inevitably lull you into the false belief that everything is all right. But as you will see, there is a lot more to genuine health than just a few chemicals, as vitamins, too, are chemicals.

The long-living never see vitamin and mineral pills and capsules; they get everything as God (or Nature) created it.

Vitamin A

Fat-soluble

Area of function - maintaining healthy skin, hair, eyes, teeth, and the lining of the mouth, throat, and nose; digestive tract, immune system, healing ability, growth, fertility.

It is associated with reduced risk of cancer, which could be due, in part, to other components of the foods (vegetables, liver, etc.) consumed. Many scientists advise against taking it in the form of supplements. It is toxic in large doses.

Sources - wheat germ, beans, spinach, celery, squash, parsley, carrot, broccoli, collards, sweet potato, green pepper, seaweed, okra, apricots, peaches, cantaloupes, papaya, strawberry, watermelon, yogurt, butter, cheeses, eggs, most fish and liver.

Vitamin B-1 (thiamine)

Area of function - carbohydrate metabolism, appetite, digestion, nervous
system, protein production, immune system.
Sources - whole grains, dried beans, lentils, peas, parsley, watercress, lettuce, sprouts, kelp, potato, almonds, milk, yogurt, yeast, fish,
mussels, oysters, organ meat (liver, kidney), lean meat.

Vitamin B-2 (riboflavin)

Areas of function - supplying oxygen for the cells, better mental capacity,
detoxification of the system, fat, carbohydrate and protein
metabolism.
Sources - all mentioned under B-1 and A.

Vitamin B-3 (niacin)

Area of function - sugar and starch metabolism, cell respiration, good
memory, digestion, maintaining healthy skin.
Sources - whole grains, bran, wheat germ, buckwheat, beans, lentils, peas,
soybean, artichoke, asparagus, okra, alfalfa, watercress,
mushroom, broccoli, peanuts, almonds, apricots, melons, organ
meat, lean meat, mussels, salmon, herring, yogurt.

Vitamin B-6 (pyridoxine)

Area of function - fat, carbohydrate and protein metabolism, preventing
complications of pregnancy and premenstrual discomfort, treating childhood mental illness.
In large doses (as supplements) may have ill-effects in people with ulcers,
in nursing mothers, or in anyone if taken with tryptophan.
Sources - whole grains, wheat germ, cabbage, green peppers, peas, nuts,
honey, eggs, avocados, bananas, organ meat.

Folic acid (folate)

Area of function - maintaining healthy bone marrow, producing red blood cells, hair, fingernails, improving the immune system and mental health.

People on drugs for epileptic treatment and cancer patients are advised by experts not to take large doses as a supplement.

Sources - whole grains, beans, lentils, peas, wheat germ, green leafy vegetables, watercress, asparagus, broccoli, peanuts, almonds, lettuce, avocados, oranges, tangerines, apricots, coconuts, romaine, sweet corn, dates, yogurt, kefir, cheese, buttermilk, organ meats.

Biotin

Area of function - processing and utilizing proteins, fatty acids and carbohydrates; nervous system, reproductive tract, skin.

Excessive amounts of raw eggs and eggnog destroy this member of the Vitamin B family, causing depression and possibly other illnesses.

Sources - whole grains, wheat germ, cauliflower, corn, mushrooms, nuts and seeds, yogurt, fish roe, oysters, salmon, cooked eggs (raw egg-white does the harm), organ meat, lean meat.

Choline

Area of function - growth and development, treating neurological disorders, lowering blood pressure, preventing heart diseases and the hardening of blood vessels, helping the liver in processing fat in case of a diet high in fat and protein.

Toxic in large doses.

Sources - whole grains, yeast, beans, lentils, peas, soybean, wheat germ, spinach, eggs, fish, fish roe, poultry, organ meat.

Let us stop here for a moment and recall this important part of the diet of the long-living. They do not get much of the second half of the list (eggs, meats); whole grains and vegetables are eaten literally every day for breakfast, for lunch, and for dinner. They do not mind eating leftovers. And indeed, they have strong heart, strong blood vessels, good nerves and memory, healthy skin, and they are slim (choline helps burn fat). *Ointments may make you look young on the outside for a short while, but with good dietary habits, you stay young inside, too - and for a long time!*

Inositol

Area of function - nerve conduction, lowering cholesterol level, helping the liver resist damage by fatty acids and toxins - just like choline.

Inositol-rich diet in experiments improved nerve conduction, but inositol taken as supplement did not! *Does this tell you something about supplements?* Caffeine destroys it. Coffee and soda guzzlers hurt themselves in many ways.

Sources - whole grains, wheat germ, beans, lentils, peas, soybean, nuts, melons, grapefruit.

PABA (para-aminobenzoic)

The body turns it easily into folic acid, another member of the Vitamin B family, so many scientists do not view PABA as another vitamin. Toxic in large doses.

Area of function - protection against grey hair, ultraviolet light and ozone; treating skin desease.

Sources - see other vitamin B sources.

Pantothenate (pantothenic acid)

Area of function - cellular metabolism, assistance in controlling and coordinating bodily functions in stress situations (e.g. sports, making love, and the regular daily activities of "civilized man".)

Sources - whole grains, bran, beans, lentils, peas, soybean, nuts and seeds, chickpeas, mushrooms, broccoli, cauliflower, cabbage, kale, molasses, queen bee jelly, fruits, yogurt, milk, eggs, salmon, chicken, turkey, organ meats.

Vitamin B-12 (cobalamin)

Area of function - maintaining healthy bone marrow; red blood cell production, immune system, mental health, digestion.

Sources - the richest sources are organ meats, less can be found in yogurt, fish, fish roe, whole grains, eggs, seeweed.

Vitamin C (ascorbic acid)

Area of function - repairing damaged cells, maintaining strong cell and blood vessel walls, building bones and teeth, promoting absorption and use of iron, protecting cells from damaging oxidation, strengthening the immune system, (possibly) lowering cholesterol levels.

Epidemiological studies have shown that people in different countries living on diet rich in fresh fruits and vegetables, have a lower risk of cancer, especially gastric and esophageal cancers. In laboratories, ascorbic acid supplements inhibited the formation of some carcinogenic compounds, but did not stop known carcinogens from inducing cancer. *It seems certain that unprocessed fruits and vegetables, with their combined vitamin, mineral and fiber content, prevent cancer.*

Sources - most fruits, especially citrus fruits, cantaloupes, strawberries, most vegetables, particularly *green and red bell peppers*, cauliflower, kale, Brussel sprouts, bean sprouts, tomatoes, potatoes, cabbage, parsley, rose hips.

Like most vitamins, vitamin C is easily destroyed if exposed to light or prolonged soaking or cooking. Eat fruits and vegetables fresh or as close to fresh as possible. Keep them covered in a cool place if you have to store them. Do not be obsessive about it, though; remember that many centenarians spend entire winters without anything fresh.

Vitamin D
Fat-soluble
Area of function - promoting strong bones and teeth, regulating the level
of calcium and phosphorus in the blood.
Highly toxic in large amounts.
Sources - produced in the skin with the presence of enough sunlight, or
can be obtained from fish roe, fish liver oil, fatty fish, liver, eggs,
butter.

Vitamin E (alpha-tocopherol)
Fat-soluble
Area of function - protection against oxidation of fatty acids that cells
badly need (cells contain fatty acids, and their oxidation is
suspected by scientists to be a major cause of many diseases and
the aging process); strengthening the immune system, protection
against pollutants and radiation - again, by inhibiting oxidation.
Sources - wheat germ, nuts and seeds, eggs, cheese, sardines and other
fish, organ meat.

Vitamin K
Fat-soluble
Area of function - normal blood clotting.
Sources - green leafy vegetables, such as spinach, cauliflower, parsley,
cabbage, mint, and seaweed.

Minerals the Body Has to Have

Calcium

Area of function - building and maintaining strong bones and teeth
(together with vitamin D and phosphorus), helping normal blood

clotting, proper functioning of nerves and muscles.

This mineral is the main structural element in the bones and teeth. Since many elderly (primarily women) suffer from osteoporosis (softening of the bones), there is a calcium-supplementing hysteria going on. Many are drinking large amounts of milk or taking high doses of calcium supplements to prevent bone loss. Here again, the natural way proves to be the best. Calcium is not absorbed if the body does not have the right amount of phosphorus and vitamin D; and notably again, people in different parts of the world, whose calcium intake is lower than the U.S. average (but is derived predominantly from vegetables), simply never suffer from this disorder. The diet of the long-living seldom includes the amount of milk we have in front of us every morning; instead, they eat lots of fruit and vegetables.

Indeed, it has been proven scientifically that there is no direct relationship between higher calcium consumption and thick bones. Excessive calcium can be harmful by accumulating in the kidneys. More over, it has been documented that *calcium supplements seem to prevent the absorption of manganese, another contributor to strong bones.*

Your system simply does not understand what the limestone crumbs are doing in your intestines. Most of them do not even dissolve fast enough to do any good (or bad, thank God). Still, many doctors (and pharmaceutical companies, of course) heartily recommend them. Consequently, consumers purchase useless (and very likely damaging) calcium supplements for a quarter billion (!) dollars annually. Does it tell you something about those who are recommending (and selling) you many other supplements? (By the way, vitamin and mineral supplements generate 3 billion dollars annually for those who are in that "business"; of course, they will do everything to "let you know": more is better.)

Other factors (very likely several components of a natural, diverse diet and physical activity) should be credited with promoting healthy bones.
We ought to mention here that too much phosphorus found in meat, most processed foods, and in most soft drinks prevents utilization of calcium. Soda addicts hurt themselves particularly because of the massive amounts of phosphate they receive through drinking several soft drinks every day (even if they are the "health protecting", "diet" type).

Eating meat daily and taking bran as fiber supplement (the new fad), drastically reduce calcium absorption. First, we simply do not need meat every day; second, getting fiber through fruits and vegetables is better as the vitamin C in them strongly enhances calcium absorption. Here again the naturally balanced diet prevails.

Sources - mother's milk and cow's milk (calcium-phosphorus ratio in them comes close to the 1:1 optimum, 2.4:1 and 1.2:1 respectively, as opposed to the 1:20 ratio in meats we consume so much of), yogurt, kefir, soups made of animal bones, eggyolk, broccoli, kale, collard, mustard and turnip greens, tubers and beans, soybean, lentils, peas, whole grains, nuts, seaweed.

The futility of the attempts to fight osteoporosis by using calcium supplements (or just simply drinking more milk) clearly demonstrates how complex and delicate the bodily functions are. Taking a few pills will not mend your health, it will only result in a patchwork. Why not have a "brand new" health? With a little bit of awareness you can easily defend your most valuable asset, despite the penetrating influence of television commercials, fellow sinners and your own long-practiced, bad habits. *And that is what this guide is all about: increasing awareness.*

Chromium

Area of function - balancing the blood sugar level, lowering the blood cholesterol level, preventing fatty deposits in blood vessels.

There is no need for more explanation as to how important this mineral is. *You ought to know that good sources of chromium (whole grains, sugars, potatoes) are almost completely depleted during processing. To make things worse, they have to rob your body of its precious chromium reserves while being digested since the process requires a certain amount of this mineral.* The long-living do not eat refined food, so chromium is another contributing element to longevity that they are not lacking in their regimen. We should be smart enough to copy them. This is the only way to do it. They have proven it to us.

Sources - whole grains (except rye), blackstrap molasses, nuts, brewer's yeast, liver, black pepper, sea food, meat.

Copper

Area of function - turning iron into hemoglobin, helping the body utilize vitamin C, promoting formation of red blood cells (if accompanied by other minerals: chromium, zink, iodine, cobalt).

Toxic in large amounts.

Sources - beans, lentils, peas, mushrooms, nuts, seafood, liver and other organ meats.

Fluoride (fluorine)

The only known benefit of fluoride consumption is (allegedly) better teeth. There is mounting evidence that it does more harm to the body than good. Most European countries have outlawed its use in water supply. We are guzzling a fair amount of a chemical that is increasing the risk of birth defects, heart disease and cancer - according to the Library of Congress Research Service. It is suspected of causing about 10,000 deaths annually in this country.

Nobody seems to care. Try to drink clear water - just in case.
Sources - seaweed, bones, tea, and water.

Iodine

Area of function - producing hormones, utilizing proteins and fats,
stimulating the circulatory system.
Sources - sea food, seaweed, and iodized salt, most fruits and vegetables,
bread.
It is simply unnecessary to use iodized salt, since far more than the trace
amount we need is in an average diet.

Iron

Area of function - main component of hemoglobin in the blood (oxygen
carrier).
Epidemiological evidences suggest that iron deficiency can cause cancer
of the stomach and the esophagus. The presence of vitamin C
boosts iron absorption, while phosphorus and chemical preservatives tend to prevent it. Our need for iron is far smaller than
many claim it to be, because the body is smart enough to re-use
it.
Vitamin C in excess destroys vitamin B-12; an adequate amount of iron
protects B-12 against C, but if there is more than necessary, it
joins vitamin C in its destructive activities. It is another good
example of the fragile balances among the constituents of the
human body, and another good reason to emulate the life-style of
the centenarians.
Excessive iron can cause impotence, frigidity, dangerous bacterium
growth, diabetes, and liver cancer. 18 mg of iron per day is
"recommended" for pregnant and lactating women. The body
recycles most of the iron, so the need is probably far less. Since
millions of women live in good health and have given life to
healthy babies without supplements, we advise you to follow the

example of the long-living: get this element, too, the natural way, through food.

Sources - beans, peas, dark-green leafy vegetables, potatoes, fruits, whole grains, blackstrap molasses, liver, kidney, heart, lean meat, shellfish, egg yolk.

Magnesium

Area of function - almost all of our cells depend on magnesium in their formation and functioning.

Magnesium is especially important for cells forming bones, muscles and nerves. *There should be a delicate balance between this mineral and calcium in order to do their job.* Magnesium deficiency causes headaches, insomnia, fatigue, heartbeat disturbances, deterioration of the heart and other muscles, skin, teeth, and kidneys. Vitamin B-6 is utilized by the body only if magnesium is present.

Toxic in large doses.

Sources - whole grains, peanuts, almond, soybeans, wheat germ, brewer's yeast, beans, lentils, peas, most dark-green vegetables, corn, apricots, bananas, blackstrap molasses, milk. Meats are poor sources, except for shellfish.

Manganese

Area of function - nervous system; should be present at protein and nucleic acid production; promotes insulin and vitamin B-1 utilization, and strong bones.

Toxic in large doses.

Sources - whole grains, beans, lentils, peas, nuts, wheat germ, tea, blueberries, ginger, sage, leafy vegetables, fruits, and wines.

Molybdenum

Area of function - utilization of fatty acids; urine formation, enzyme
systems.

Toxic in large doses.

Epidemiological evidences (in some areas of China, the U.S.A. and
Africa) link molybdenum deficiency to cancer of the esophagus.

Sources - beans, lentils, peas, soybeans, leafy vegetables, whole grains,
organ meat, yeast.

Phosphorus

Area of function - forming strong bones and teeth, all the processes
involving utilization and transformation of substances in the
body.

As it was mentioned before (see Calcium), optimum utilization of
phosphorus and calcium is possible only if the optimum balance
between the two is maintained. *Excessive phosphorus levels
inhibit calcium absorption, which will result in bone loss.*

*Through processed foods and "manufactured" drinks, the phosphorus intake
of an average American is extremely high - and getting even higher.*
Phosphorus compounds (phosphates) widely used as additives
and preservatives in the mentioned foods and drinks seem to be
even more aggressive in "calcium flushing" than the naturally
occuring phosphorus.

In laboratory experiments, changing from natural, unprocessed to
"normal", supermarket foods doubled the phosphorus intake of
volunteers, resulting in intestinal distress, soft stool, lower calcium levels in blood, higher levels in stool samples (indicating
bone loss) - in the course of four short weeks. No more comments.

Sources - processed foods, most soft drinks, meat, fish, eggs, bran, wheat
germ, beans, lentils, peas, nuts.

Potassium

Area of function - proper muscle and nerve functions, regulating fluid
balances in cells.

Toxic even in small quantities taken as supplement. Some managed to
get ulcers this way.
Sources - fresh fruits (mainly bananas, oranges, grapefruit), peanuts, nuts,
squash, broccoli, wheat germ, potatoes.

Selenium

Area of function - enzyme systems, oxygen and energy transfer, producing
nucleic acids, antibodies, sperm, maintenance of muscle and red
blood cells, skin, nails, and hair, protecting cells against oxidation.
*Epidemiological studies and laboratory experiments indicate that selenium
protects against cancers, blood vessel disease, heart disease and the
toxicity of heavy metals.* It also seems likely that *selenium
deficiency*, if combined with a diet rich in polyunsaturated (!) fat,
promotes cancer growth.
Toxic in larger doses.
Sources - whole grains, vegetables, garlic, fruits, nuts, brewer's yeast,
seafood, liver and other organ meats.

Silicon

Area of function - proper growth, embrionic development, regulating
nutrient and water transfer, healing wounds and ulcers, building
strong bones.
At younger ages, the blood vessels contain high levels of silicon, which will
decline with aging. High concentrations of this mineral in drinking water has been shown to protect against heart disease. Some
researchers consider it the active element of dietary fiber. One
more reason to avoid processed foods which are lacking fiber.
Sources - (unless removed during processing) most natural foods offer

ample supply, except for meats (but bones and skin are rich in silicon).

Sodium

Area of function - participates in the formation of the digestive juices, regulates the movement of nutrients and fluids through the cell walls.

3 to 5 mg per day is considered safe; larger amounts contribute to high blood pressure, a major cause of heart attacks and strokes. Most processed foods have far too much salt in them as preservative or "taste enhancer". Another reason to avoid them.

Zinc

Area of function - essential for insulin production and for more than 100 enzymes, the nucleic acids, cell production and repair, wound healing, normal growth, prevention of anemia.

High concentrations of zinc seem to offset the protective effect of selenium against certain cancers, but efficiently suppressed some other cancers in animal experiments. It offers protection against the toxicity of lead and cadmium.

Sources - whole grains, beans, lentils, peas, brewer's yeast, corn, carrots, millet, lentils, yams, peanuts, nuts, shellfish, organ meat, milk, eggs.

There are some other minerals (tin, sulfur, vanadium, etc.) suspected of playing some beneficial role in the human body, but, since they are present in minute quantities, their research is very difficult.

On the other hand, what little we know about some others: cadmium, arsenic, beryllium, nickel, and lead, suggests that they are *contributing factors to cancer* at several sites (the mouth, the esophagus, the large intestine, the larynx, the lungs, the breasts in females, and the bladder); at least *this is what the analyses of the water supplies show in 10 river basins of the U.S.* In minute quantities, they offer some physiological benefits. Almost any kind of diet will supply the trace amounts we need.

There can be an infinite number of combinations of and interactions between vitamins, minerals, drugs, alcohol, foods and food additives in your body. Some of these interactions are well-known to scientists. So, if you are drinking alcohol, or taking vitamin or mineral supplements or prescribed drugs, always ask your doctor about their possible (side) effects on other vitamins or minerals.

Always try not to interfere with the natural processes of your body; resort to prescribed drugs or any supplements only if it is really necessary and recommended by someone experienced and knowledgeable, like your doctor. When it comes to your health, never listen to anyone who is trying to sell you something, no matter how great the "new breakthrough" sounds. It is better to read about it, and when armored with some of your own knowledge, talk it over with your doctor.

A recent introduction of a drug, called Lovastatin (trade name: Mevacor), is a good example of how scientific breakthroughs work. The new pill, at a cost of $1000-$3000 per year, will lower the cholesterol in the veins of about 20 million Americans with already dangerously high levels. Probably many more will be tempted to use the same drug as a preventive shortcut. A billion dollar gold mine for the manufacturer.

Sober-minded experts have already cautioned that Lovastatin is not an alternative to a healthy diet. There are many reasons for that. For many people *diet low in cholesterol is the only effective way to bring down cholesterol to the normal level*. The body itself needs and produces a considerable amount of cholesterol, more than one can take in with almost any diet.

The new drug forces the liver to produce less cholesterol, so the liver will remove the needed amount from the blood. Isn't it like causing imbalance deliberately? The drug is disturbing a normally functioning organ because the person cannot or will not eat the right food.

Due to the possibility of side-effects (cataracts and liver damage), patients are advised by the Food and Drug Administration to have blood tests every six weeks(!), and an eye examination annually.

This is how a real scientific breakthrough works. Try to imagine how "well" the "quack" breaktroughs can work. (Some are called 'revolutionary weight-loss program', some others, 'revolutionary protein formula', etc.)

Every sensible person agrees that the safest way to reduce the risk of blood vessel disease is by living on a healthy, low-fat, low-cholesterol diet. *Yes, there is more to heart disease prevention than just limiting cholesterol production.*

Food Additives

(It is a shame that we have to add this part.) By looking at the shiny boxes and bags, and the glowing bottles on the shelves of our supermarkets, we get the impression that probably never before Man had a richer and better food supply. "Rich" is unquestionably the right phrase to describe what we consume, but is it "better"? It looks better, it tastes better than what our ancestors could have ever had, nobody can deny. But consider this: *About 3000 substances (most of them manufactured chemicals) are added intentionally to the foods we consume daily.* Most of them serve as agents to prevent spoilage or to lengthen "shelf-life", but many of them are used simply to make the "product" look more attractive, or to make the manufacturing process easier.

Nothing is added without a reason, but *there are approximately 12,000 other substances that get into our food supply unintentionally during growing, handling, transporting, and processing.*

You are right if you think it is almost impossible to thoroughly test all these chemicals one by one (not to mention their combinations) for their possible negative effects on our health. First of all, the expenses would be astronomical. At least 1000 rats are needed to demonstrate the harm if an additive does that harm to 1 out of 1000 people. If there is no indication of ill-effect, some other species should be tried, and then another...and 1000 of each species...(or more?) Some substances, like arsenic, do induce cancer in humans, but not in animals. Financially and scientifically a very difficult task it is. Hence, the question is: are those "uninvited guests" in our diet properly monitored? In other words: *is our diet safe*?

If you think that our institutions responsible for the safety of the food supply are perfectly able to do the job, and they clearly see the potential danger these chemicals represent, thus, the problem of food additives is their paramount concern, then think again. In ranking the health hazards in the U.S. diet, the Food and Drug Administration (FDA) lists food additives in fifth place, below even nutrient deficiencies.

Furthermore, there is a very influencial "food industry lobby" fighting against the attempts to restrict their freedom to use thousands of known chemicals, and to invent and introduce new ones. When the FDA proposed a ban on two antibiotics routinely fed to animals, Congress rejected it under pressure from agricultural groups and pharmaceutical companies.

The constant use of antibiotics may result in resistant bacteria. The FDA has already admitted the occurrence of ailments and deaths linked to such bacteria.

This very food industry is supposed to test the additives and certify that they pose no threat to public health. Information is frequently withheld from the public; environment and consumer protection groups are not adequately represented in discussions regarding these matters of vital public interest.

In the light of all this, it is no wonder that *of thousands of food additives only a portion have been tested for their cancer-causing potential*, according to standards currently considered acceptable in the scientific community. The possibility of additional health hazards, other than cancer, and the effects of consuming small amounts of chemicals during a long period of time require more attention and more conscientious testing.

It is not easy to identify the additives in our food. Federal regulations are inconsistent; most additives simply do not have to be listed on the labels. In many cases, listing all the chemicals would be impossible (due to a lack of space on the label).

Here is a list of additives most frequently found in boxes, bags, jars and cans on the shelves of our grocery stores.

Aspartame (NutraSweet TM)

Added to soft drinks, candies, cakes, diet foods, canned fruits and juices, etc.

The commercials give you the impression that you are guzzling the safest drink on earth in the shape of a "diet" soft drink; but for your own sake, remember saccharin which was introduced in 1907, and its use was restricted a few years ago because it proved to be carcinogenic. Before 1970, it was extensively used together with cyclamates, which were then banned for the same reason.

Aspartame, in laboratory tests, caused brain damage, depression, headaches, fatigue, constipation, and menstrual irregularities. It has not been tested for carcinogenicity.

BHA (Butylated Hydroxyanisole)

One of the most common food preservatives in the U.S. It is used in dry breakfast cereals, dry sausages, frozen fresh sausages, freeze-dried meats, dry mixes for beverages and desserts, potato flakes, chewing gum base, beverages, ice cream, candy, gelatin desserts, baked goods, etc.

Several studies failed to prove BHA to be carcinogenic or mutagenic, but was found to retard growth, to cause major changes in brain chemistry of the offsprings, and to inhibit muscle contraction in other experiments. It is banned in England.

It has been discovered by scientists that BHA inhibits chemically induced cancers in animals.

BHT (Butylated Hydroxytoluene)

Widely used as a food additive in animal fats, frozen fresh sausages, dry
     breakfast cereals, potato flakes, chewing gum base, etc.
In several experiments BHT caused birth defects, cancer, and depression
     of growth, and enhanced growth of tumors in laboratory animals.
     Its use is not permitted in Australia, Sweden and England.
On the other hand, large quantities of this chemical can inhibit cancer
     growth induced by some chemicals.

Benzoic Acid (Sodium Benzoate)

Added to margarine, fruit juices, maraschino cherries, pickles, soft drinks,
     ice cream, candies, chewing gums, baked goods, fruit jellies, etc.
Most berries contain benzoic acid in its natural form. In laboratories,
     animals fed larger amounts of its manufactured form showed
     signs of brain damage, depressed growth, loss of weight, and
     neurological disorders. There were indications that acting
     together with other chemicals it can cause cancer.

Caffeine

Found in soft drinks, coffee, tea.
Its side-effects are well-known: nervousness, irritability, insomnia, and
     unnaturally high heartbeat rate. In laboratory tests it produced
     abnormal changes in cell reproduction. Nursing mothers and
     families with small children have to be particularly careful
     because caffeine works more "effectively" in children due to the
     lower body weight. *A cup of regular cola for a child is nearly the
     equivalent to four cups*(!) *of coffee for an adult.*

The caffeine's effect on the central nervous system of adults is de-
     monstrated every day, so it is a prudent assumption to say, that

caffeine is not doing any good to the developing brain and nervous system of a small child or especially of a tiny creature in the mother's womb.

Artificial Colors

Added to ice creams, candies, cakes, canned foodstuffs, baked goods, soft drinks, juices, dairy products, etc.

Since the turn of the century, dozens of chemical substances have been used as additives to foodstuffs and drinks just to make them look more attractive. Most proved harmful and are not permitted anymore. Many of them are cancer-causing agents and were banned after a "long service".

Even today the consumer is left in the dark, because manufacturers do not have to put the names of most coloring chemicals on the labels. You will find in most cases only these words: "artificial color(s) added".

Most of them are made of coal tar or petrochemicals, and *almost all of them have caused cancer or other ill-effects in laboratory animals.* Some coloring agents are made of insects.

Citrus Red No. 2 caused cancer in animal experiments, but is still used to give oranges a color "nicer" than the natural yellow.

Yellow No. 5 and No. 6 are commonly listed on labels by name. So far none of them has been associated with serious ill-effects other than allergy reactions (No. 5), and eye defects and blindness (No. 6) in test animals.

Red No. 40 has limited use in baked products; in some experiments it caused cancer in mice.

Artificial Flavors

Added to candy, ice cream, ice, syrups, pudding, baked goods, pickles, meat products, margarine, dairy products, breakfast cereals, soups, drinks, etc.

Manufactured mainly from petrochemicals, well over 1500 artificial food flavorings are currently in use in the U.S. *Most of them have not been tested sufficiently for possible health hazards; some of them have not been tested at all.*

The names of artificial flavors are not disclosed on food labels. What is more, the composition of many of them are treated as "trade secrets", and there is very limited access to information on these compounds or the test results when they are tested.

Especially children are exposed to large quantities through consuming soft drinks, candy, ice cream, cookies, etc.

Remember coumarin and safrole (after long use both were found carcinogenic, and consequently banned), and try to stay away from products laced with artificial flavors.

Carrageenan (Irish Moss)

Used in fruit juices, cakes, ice cream, cheeses, soups, beer, wine, chocolate drinks, sausages, canned meats, marshmallows, pet foods, etc.

This seaweed has been an important food additive in America and Europe for centuries. Relatively recent studies have revealed, that it causes cancer, ulcers, inflammation, liver damage, depressed growth, and birth defects in laboratory animals.

Sodium (or Potassium) Nitrate and Sodium Nitrite

Used in cured meat and meat products.

Both occur naturally in vegetables as well. In certain circumstances, they can combine with amines, *creating the very potent cancer-causing nitrosamins. Vitamin C, which is present in vegetables, and vitamin E seem to effectively inhibit this process.*

Cured meats are "rich sources" of nitrates and nitrites; even *preformed* nitrosamins can be found in them (especially in bacon).

Monosodium Glutamate (MSG)

Added to about ten thousand processed foods. It is extracted from wheat or corn gluten or sugar-beets. As a "flavor enhancer", it is the most extensively applied food additive in the U.S.

It has been shown that it causes eye damage, brain lesions, stunted skeletal development, female sterility, and obesity in laboratory animals. As for humans, about one quarter of the population experience allergic reactions when exposed to "normal levels" of MSG. This is the so-called Chinese Restaurant Syndrome.

Hydrolized (Vegetable) Protein

It replaced MSG in baby foods for a while, but it is still added to gourmet foods, canned tuna, etc.

This substance is very similar to MSG, and has been found to cause brain damage in infant mice.

Modified Starch

Added to baby food, cream fillings, pie fillings, drinks, gourmet foods, sauces, gravies, soups, spaghetti sauce, etc.

It is not considered harmful, but it adds empty calories to the diet, since fiber, vitamins, proteins, minerals, and enzymes are almost totally missing from it.

Hydrogenated Oil (or "Partially" Hydrogenated)

Used in margarines, baked goods, candy, dry drink mixes, peanut butter, and hundreds more; also used extensively in restaurants.

Extracted by chemicals, deodorized, heated, pushed through a mesh in *hydrogen, vegetable oils are "manufactured" into a white, tasteless, odorless fat completely void of all vitamins and minerals. Essential fatty acids are either destroyed or distorted. The resulting abnormal fatty acids can cause heart disease, arteriosclerosis, cancer, high blood cholesterol levels, neurological and skin diseases, arthritis, etc.*

If artificial flavors, articificial colors, and artificial preservatives are added, it is called margarine. This "stuff" has been heavily advertised as healthy, since it is made of healthy vegetable oils. It is a big moneymaker for many companies. Americans consume billions of pounds of this fat every year. **Do not even touch it!**

Try to avoid anything that has "partially" hydrogenated vegetable (or coconut or palm) oil in it.

Propionates and Sorbates

Used in bakery products, chocolate, fruit jellies and preserves, pizza crust, poultry stuffing, cheeses, etc.

Both occur in nature, but the amounts intentionally added to our food are manufactured in factories. Propionates are known to possess no major health threatening properties. They inhibit the growth of certain bacteria and molds.

Before harvest some molds invade certain crops: mainly peanuts, corn, and cottonseed, and to a much lesser degree: walnuts, pistachios, almonds, and pecans. Occasionally, a substance called Alfatoxin is produced by them, which is one of the most powerful cancer-causing agents known. Try to avoid raw peanuts.

EDTA

Added to canned seafood, mushrooms, pickled cucumber and cabbage, beer, liquor, salad dressing, sandwich spread, mayonnaise, potato salad, etc.

It is eliminated from the body rapidly without absorption. The reason for concern is that it flushes out vital minerals, adding to the deficiencies an unsuspecting person is suffering from anyway due to the consumption of overprocessed foods. It is another good reason for pregnant women (and for all) to read the labels and to stay away from alcohol.

Glycerides

Added to commercial baked goods, non-dairy cream substitutes, oils, desserts, etc.
Processed by the body as fat; considered safe.

THE FOOD WE EAT - THE WAY WE LIVE

Thinking of health or especially long life, it inevitably comes to one's mind: what could be the kind of food (or the single factor) that makes an unusually long life span possible. Having looked at the life-style of the long-living peoples of the world, it seems clear and obvious that not a single thing but a lucky coincidence of several factors is the "secret" in their longevity and vigorous health. They eat the right things, drink the right things and live the right way - because they have had no alternative. We in the affluent societies have all the alternatives in the world.

We have been yielding to the temptations of civiliation so much and for so long, that we seem to have forgotten the good old ways. In our ignorance we are being choked to death by the very wealth we have and our ancestors had worked so hard to create. Do not feel offended by the word "ignorance", for even the best doctors, the cream of the trade, just looked on dumbfoundedly when the diseases of civilization walked in through the back door. We would love to believe that today they know how to prevent them - because they certainly cannot cure them.

Prevention and possibly reversal is the point here. The unshakeable proof is embodied in the longevious peoples. The common factors in their diets and life-styles are the only dependable guidelines for us towards one hundred happy years.

Let us see now what we eat when we eat. In a relatively short form we attempt to present what the long-living peoples and the latest scientific discoveries can teach us about the major food groups.

Animal Supplied Foods

Red meat, organ meats, wild game, poulty, shellfish and fin fish, bones, eggs, dairy products.

As you already know, the long-living have not had access to much meat in general; in fact, meat is considered a delicacy on their table on special occasions, but the most frequently on the weekends. Their "meaty" days mean red meat or poultry, which happen to be less healthy than fin fish for instance, but there is no chance or temptation to eat too much. Thick bones are wisely utilized in all kinds of soups, with all the minerals in them. Eggs are scarce; one or two a day are shared by the whole family in noodles, cakes, or other meals.

As far as dairy products are concerned, their scarcity helps them in that case too. The people in Vilcabamba and Hunza consume little dairy products, the people of the Caucasus eat and drink more. But "luckily" again for the latter folks, there are no supermarkets there, so they have to settle for whatever amount of milk their animals produce.

The potentially harmful part is the fat (or cream); it is only a small part of the milk, which is (like the few eggs) shared by the whole family. The rest of the milk is then turned into low-fat farmers cheese, cottage cheese, cheese, kefir, and yogurt. The latter products happen to be very healthy; you can eat them by the pound, it will not hurt you. And they do eat them by the pound (just like the Masai in Africa), lowering blood cholesterol levels, strengthening their bones and muscles, preventing heart disease - without having any idea about the great service they are doing for their health.

What is wrong with meat? We are eating our "fellow creatures", so it is supposed to have everything we need from vitamins to minerals, from proteins to fat. Indeed, red meat, poultry, organ meats, and fishes have virtually all the nutrients we humans need.

Keep in mind that there is a great deal of "overlapping" between animal supplied foods and the ones plants give us. The long-living people are a very good example of this, since most of them live on near-vegetarian diets that afford them excellent health.

Animals provide us with concentrates of fat, protein, cholesterol, vitamins, minerals, amino acids, etc. They are just "too good" for us. It is easy to consume too much of the good stuff. We were not created for that.

Fat, protein and cholesterol in meats and dairy products (fatty cheeses, cream) are likely to do harm if consumed in large quantities. *Protein is stored as fat if not used up immediately by the body, so even the leanest meat can make you fat.*

Lower total calorie intake inhibits the incidence of life-threatening diseases (heart and blood vessel diseases, cancer) and significantly increases life span.

Indeed, the average calorie intake of the longevious peoples is around 1200 to 1800 (in some areas 2000 - 2500) calories a day, about half the U.S. average. **Overweight people simply do not live long.**

High dietary fat intake (saturated or unsaturated) is a major contributor to cancer (mainly breast, colon and prostate), and blood vessel diseases (heart attacks and strokes).

At lower levels of fat consumption, polyunsaturated fats seem to be more active in causing cancer than at higher (total) levels.

What a "lucky" coincidence: those long-living folks cook with the "worst" kind of saturated fats (lard, tallow), but use just a very small amount every day. On the other hand, the "civilized man" thinks that eating bacon, hamburgers, sandwiches, fish, steak, eggs, cheese, fried potatoes every day is absolutely necessary for a "well-balanced" diet. Since these meals contain or are soaked with fat (and cholesterol), and are lacking vital nutrients, they simply kill the "civilized man".

No matter how well-prepared you are at selecting the right vegetable oil or fish oil (the new fad), if you eat our "normal" food too frequently, your stomach cannot have room for the right meals, so you are doomed.

This year too, about 1,300,000 individuals in the U.S. will die of heart attacks, strokes and cancer by New Year's Eve. Close to one million of them could have celebrated many more New Year's Eves, if only they had made a few sensible changes in their life - *but by now they do not have a chance. Up to 90% of these tragedies are self-inflicted.*

Do not be misled by your body weight: there are less overweight people proportionally in Finland than in the U.S., still they have the highest heart attack rate in the world. *Concentrating on diets promising*

weight-loss through lower calorie intake, is a job less than halfway done.
A diet has to comprise good food not just little food.

There is a way to take advantage of animal supplied foods. Eat the ones that have valuable components but not harmful ones. The long-living peoples cook soups of bones with some meat on them, with lots of vegetables, and eat large amounts of yogurt and low-fat cheeses. (In the case of the long-living, "large amount" always means moderate by our standards!) At any rate, these are foods you just cannot eat too much of.

Beef is the hardest meat to digest; fin fish is the easiest, according to the degree of fat saturation - with the other kinds in between. *Cooking methods can diminish the difference. Try to avoid anything fried.* Broiling/barbecuing is better, but bad enough; boiling is the best. The first two methods create significant amounts of carcinogenic substances.

Processed meats invariably contain preservatives that cause cancer. Among people, like the ones we have studied here, who consume little meat, fat, eggs and unfermented milk, heart disease and cancer are virtually unknown, except at very old ages.

Plant Supplied Foods

Vegetables, grains, fruits, nuts, berries, and herbs.

They can provide basically everything animal supplied foods do, except for cholesterol. The peoples of the Caucasus, Hunza and Vil-cabamba do not suffer from malnutrition despite their primary dependance on plant supplied foods. Actually, they do better than any other group in the world. Why? The chief reason is that **their diet does not promote cancers, heart attacks, strokes, diabetes, etc. as does ours, but on the contrary: it helps the body reach the life span it was designed for.** Their diet, combined with their active life-style, is the only remedy for the plagues we seem to be cursed with.

There is one component in the plants whose importance cannot be emphasized enough: **it is fiber.** If you really want to find the "secret" of human longevity, fiber should be it. It seems to be a paradox that something we cannot even digest is " the secret". But it is; you can bet your life on it. Never forget this; your life depends on it.

In places like the ones we have studied, where people consume fiber-rich foods, mainly unprocessed vegetables, whole-grains, and fruits, virtually absent are what we know as "civilization diseases": heart disease, strokes, cancers, obesity, ulcers, varicose veins, diabetes, cavities, constipation, digestive discomfort, appendicitis, and diverticulitis.

Of course, it is not the rough, undigestible material that makes their bodies grow, move or function in any way, but the vitamins, minerals, protein and energy sources the fiber carries. These are the substances the "civilized man" is getting through crystal clear sugar, over-purified flour, and countless supplements and "scientific formulas".

But it is not the same. It is just like trying to steer the wheels of a car assembled from shiny, "perfected" parts, desperately lubricating it with newer and newer lubricants (even the seats and the brake pads - just in case). It will not work. The new parts just do not fit the basic design, even though they are "perfected" to do the job. We cannot change the basic design that took four billion years to get as good as it is.

Nevertheless, the affluent societies just keep on trying. The U.S. is the leading sinner with the consumption of about 120 pounds of pure white sugar, the same amount of pure white flour, 5 pounds of food additives (many of them obscure chemicals or known cancer-causing agents) for every person (even babies included), every year.

These are incredibly high amounts, considering the fact that the body does not need even a tiny bit of them. What is more, it does not know how to handle them. *"Manufactured" foods disrupt delicate balances, causing the malfunction of organs and the whole system.* As a result, sometimes too much of something is produced (cells, in case of a cancer), or not enough (insulin, in case of diabetes) - just to mention two imbalances.

The ways of the human body are so complicated, that scientists are unable to explain exactly how and why civilization diseases occur. They can, of course, see the connection between certain malfunctions and substances.

Researchers in many countries found close correlation between concentrated carbohydrates (white sugar and white flour) and cancer. It is very hard to determine how much a certain substance affects the population, because generally who eats white sugar, eats white flour, and meat, and fat, and cream, etc.

It is well documented that as new nations take over the "civilized" diet, after about twenty to thirty years of "grace period", our civilization diseases strike them, too. They do not even have to have two cars in every family; the new diet itself can do the "job".

This is what is happening in many parts of the world. In Eastern Europe or the Middle East, for instance, now, with the "grace period" over, people are dumbfounded by the increasing number of (mainly younger) people dying of heart attacks, strokes, diabetes, cancer etc. The real problem is that they do not even know why they are dying, since these things are new to them.

It seems, however, that nobody can catch up with us here in the U.S., as far as dying is concerned. *The U.S. is among the world leaders in heart diseases, strokes, cancers, and diabetes.* Most of these diseases started reaching epidemic proportions after the turn of the century in the affluent societies. The first diagnosed heart attack took place around 1910. Since then, the life expectancy of a 45-year-old person in the U.S. has increased by only two years. The higher survival rate of babies is the sole contributor to the increase of the average life span.

White sugar and white flour are powders of energy. These concentrates are probably worse than meat or fat, because they are almost completely void of any nutritional value, and many times our taste buds just cannot resist them. Refined carbohydrates deplete the body's vitamin and mineral reserves, leading to cancer, diabetes, blood vessel disease, osteoporosis, tooth decay, and all the unpredictable consequencies.

When not processed, all plant supplied foods contain fiber. *The presence of this "useless" bulk seems to have many benefits.* It simply does what it is "supposed" to do, or rather, what one could expect from a natural diet: it helps maintain those delicate balances we have just talked about. Fiber makes the bowel movement regular, smooth and fast. It helps the body get rid of excessive fat, cholesterol, harmful bacteria and other toxic and cancer-causing substances. It lowers blood pressure and blood cholesterol levels, slows down and regulates the absorption of nutrients, preventing a shock-effect on the organs. It even "knows" how to stimulate the production of the "good" cholesterol, HDL (which inhibits the clogging of veins) and how to reduce the level of "bad" cholesterol, LDL (which promotes it).

Indeed, a fiber-rich diet can cure adult onset diabetes (90% of all diabetics); it can reduce the insulin need for the rest of the patients by as much as 38 % (consult your doctor !). It can also rejuvenate clogged blood vessels around the heart, in the legs, and the brain. Hypoglycemia (low blood sugar level), constipation, hemorrhoids, heartburn and digestive discomfort are remedied by a high-fiber diet normally in a matter of days or weeks. Relieving constipation with bulky food is the only way to prevent appendicitis and diverticulosis (small pockets pouching out of the large intestine). *Do not cheat yourself with laxatives.*

People living on fiber-rich diets, have never been afflicted with these problems; not bad for something that is free and can cure or prevent all these diseases.

Since fiber adds to the feeling of fullness, and drops the insulin level - which, in turn, reduces appetite - the *natural* diet cures obesity, and helps control weight, as well. Moreover, fiber helps the body get rid of the extra fat through the bowel movement, and not all the calories in fiber-rich foods are absorbed. The same diet ensures the balance of minerals, thus preventing the women's dreaded disease: osteoporosis.

Those who eat fiber-rich foods, normally eat less meat, fat, and unprocessed foods; thereby, they can maintain healthy acid levels and can prevent or even cure ulcers.

You might think that this fiber story sounds like a cure-all treatment. Well, it almost is. Nature or God did not make our ancestors look for good food in vain during 4 billion years.

Besides fats, meat, white sugar, white flour and additives, **vegetable oils** *represent another major threat to the health of the public.* If processed at high temperature, these oils lose their nutritional value for us. Since most brands sold in supermarkets are not cold-pressed but extracted by chemicals, heated and then treated by chemicals, they should be avoided. What is more, if overheated, vegetable oils become carcinogenic. Margarines, after having gone through the process of hydrogenation (artificial flavors and preservatives are added, as well), are totally useless, and do more harm than good.

Let us mention a group of plant supplied foods that, aside from their nutritional value, have even some *medical virtues*.

Garlic is very popular all over the world, known to promote lower blood cholesterol, blood sugar, and blood pressure; it also protects against or inhibits cancer, arteriosclerosis, stomach ulcers, vaginal infections, and meningitis (caused by fungi). It is a natural detoxifier. Garlic is effective only in its natural, "smelly" form, so there are no shortcuts; do not waste your money on "garlic oil". The long-living people use garlic in almost everything they eat. You should do the same as much as you can! Eat it raw in the evening at least once a week when you have no company, or use it in soups. Eating a mint leaf will also help cover up smell.

Honey has vitamins, minerals and proteins in minute quantities. It contains mainly simple sugars, so do not see it as a substitute for white sugar. Buy only the dark, natural, uncooked, unprocessed kind. Keep always honey at home; eat it every day (in yogurt, cottage cheese, tea, etc.). Use it sparingly, not more than a teaspoon a day.

Teas made of chamomile, hyssop, linden flowers, mullein, peppermint, rose hips, and uva ursi. These plants have been used for centuries for digestive disturbances and related complaints, minor colds, cramps, sore throat, etc. Do not expect great results, but one or two cups might ease your discomfort. Avoid larger quantities. As for the numerous other herbs, if you wish to get acquainted with them, please, read books that show restraint in recommending herbs as a remedy for different diseases. Some of them can be outright dangerous or even fatal.

Seeds and **Nuts** are extremely beneficial sources of vitamins, minerals, fats, fiber, and some essential amino acids not available in many plants. A handful for a snack is enough for a day, as they are high in calories.

Alcohol and Smoking

Studies conducted in several countries of the world have shown a direct relationship between alcohol abuse and cancer, also damage to the nervous system, the liver and other organs. It seems very likely that the cancer-causing effect of alcohol is a result of vitamin and mineral deficiencies, which alcohol abusers frequently suffer from. The alcohol in homemade strong spirits seems to be the most harmful of all, but mass-produced booze also hides dozens of potentially dangerous chemicals, as well. The "manufacturers" are not required to disclose what they put into their brew.

Smoking in itself causes heart attacks, damage to blood vessels, and cancer at different sites of the body. Together with alcohol it has a powerful synergistic effect; in other words: they amplify each other's damaging effect.

The safest way is to stay away from them. Younger people and pregnant women should be especially careful with the two substances (and other drugs, of course). *A young, developing body is even more defenseless than that of a strong adult.*

The long-living people we have studied never abuse alcohol or smoking. Light homemade wine is frequently drunk but always in moderation, one to two glasses a day. *It is a prudent assumption that their wine contains less chemicals than our wines do.*

Today's World - Supplements, "Diets", Supermarkets, Fast Food

There are two types of people who are taking vitamin and mineral supplements. For those who are confused by the claims of books and ads, we recommend please, stop taking those pills. It is wasting money, and might well be harmful.

The second group is made up of those who are influenced so much by the claims regarding the alleged deficiencies of all our foods and consequently the "vital importance" of supplements, that they religiously believe in them. We do not try to change beliefs. What we recommend for both groups is to concentrate on eating and drinking the right things. We hope, after having gone through the previous chapters, it is obvious that there is more to nutrition than mere vitamins, minerals and calories.

This leads us to the so-called "diets". The honest efforts of some and the greed of many more have produced innumerable "diets". The effectiveness of these regimens are normally measured by the speed and the amount of weight-loss.

A 40-50 day fasting will almost certainly result in death. Even before the end, organs and the brain suffer some irreversible damage. *The body is in a state of emergency, nothing is working the normal way.* Most of these "diets" will not result in death; they "allow" some food and drink, which slows down the dying process. But the rapid weight-loss indicates that the "dieting" person is advancing toward death.

Of course, no "diet" expects you to die, and you will stop "dieting" probably in time anyway. O.K.,then what? What will you do next? Are you going to walk the tightrope between the regimen that results in over-weight and the "diet" that leans towards death?

There are some "extremes". Some doctors, in their pursuit of profits, give their names to "diet programs" marketed on television, claiming that you can eat everything in any quantity, gaining or losing weight is just a matter of mental state. (Or perhaps, the "miracle pills" and "protein formulas" are the real extremes?)

The large number of the "diets" is the proof that they are totally inefficient. Yes, many are effective in making you lose weight, *but they totally miss the point.* Five billion dollars are spent by people in the U.S. every year on "formulas" and "diets" to lose weight. But *losing weight is not the point*! No matter how slim you are or how slim you will become, you are not much better off than half of the U. S. population (overweight people), unless you eat the right food.

Do not put your faith in any "diet" or vitamin, mineral, or protein "formulas". *There is more to health.* Nobody, but nobody knows what your body needs. Let it do its job; it has four billion years of experience.

Eating the foods Nature devised for us and leaving out the ones we "manufacture", will afford you great health - and the excess weight will be shed, if there is any. **This is the point!** Any regimen which you cannot live on for the rest of your life, cannot do you much good. Do not jeopardize your health. Do not waste your money on fad diets, do not let them coerse you to miss the point! Try to follow the life-style of the long-living peoples we have become acquainted with in this guide. Live the way they live; eat what they eat; drink what they drink - as much as you can. *Their longevity is the proof that their regimen is* **"The Diet".** This is the only way to a sound mind in a sound body.

We have to agree that it is very hard to eat natural foods these days. Not that it is not available; it is because we are lazy. We go for the meal that is already prepared for us, and seems as good and healthy as the one we could make, if we were not busy or lazy. The sad truth is that it is not as healthy as it seems to be.

Let us walk into a typical fast food place. This is where millions of us chase away our hunger almost every day; it seems to be cheap, and it is very convenient. It is not a gross exaggeration to say, that what we call fast food today is the manifestation of everything bad the modern food industry has to offer.

A typical lunch there gives you energy equivalent to all the food a hardworking adult in Vilcabamba eats in one day. Would you think that a well-packed hamburger, large fries, and a chocolate shake "hide" more than 1200 calories? In other countries many reach older ages living on just this much, so we will never die of starvation. Besides the fat in the ground beef *(about 50% fat, like in most other meats)*, fried potato, fried chicken, fried fish, sausage, omlette, bacon, hash browns, coleslaw, cheeseburgers, etc. are all soaked with fat (30 to 80% of the calories coming from fat, as opposed to the 3 to 15 % in the diet of the long-living).

During frying, cancer-causing substances are created in the meat products and the frying fat.

Since in the eyes of most of us, meat makes a meal complete, balanced and rich, that is what we are offered everywhere every day, and that is what we eat everywhere every day. This way an average person eats over 100 grams of protein every day, about three times the amount his body would like to have. The same body would like to have meat only once a week on the average. It would not like to have sugar, excessive phosphorus, bromine, caffeine, preservatives, artificial colors, flavors, and sweeteners at all. But even young children are guzzling soft drinks. *Many do not even know what water tastes like.*

When siren voices are singing into your ears that the stuff on your plate is healthy and good for you, and that you have a whole new kind of thirst, which you should quench with their brew, it is hard to resist.

Of course, *they do not tell you* that you eat three times more protein than you need, ten to fifty times more fat than you need, and ten times less fiber than you need (2 to 3 grams a day instead of 20 to 30!). They do not tell you that the bread, the bun, and the crust are lacking almost all the bran, vitamins and minerals, without which your body cannot function properly.

You cannot blame the owners of those companies; they do not twist your child's arm; they just twist his brain; they just go for the fast buck; they just go with the profit-seeking crowd - the same way you follow the junk food seeking crowd.

If you think they care about your health, then go back to the additive section of this guide or listen to the following example. Most of us think that since saccharin has proven to be carcinogenic, it is banned. No, it is not banned; you can still buy cancer-causing saccharin in sodas, it is written on the can. Likewise, soft drinks, that promise Nature's fresh fruit juices, are made with tap water and about 10% cheap fruit juice, and a chemical called BVO (brominated vegetable oil). This substance is outlawed for such use in many European countries, because when rats were fed a diet with only one half percent BVO in it, after a short eighty days, they suffered damage to their heart, kidneys, liver, and other organs. *This is what our children are guzzling - and nobody knows or cares.*

Do you have constipation because your intestines haven't seen enough fiber for years? Smart companies are selling you laxatives, so you can make it until the onset of colon cancer. Do you have heartburn because of the deep-fried junk? Smart companies will sell you antacids, even with calcium supplement "to strengthen" the bones that a junk food diet (dirt-poor in vitamins, minerals, and fiber but filthy-rich in calories and chemicals) is making brittle.

Now, why would they tell you that a humble whole-wheat bread sandwich can easily take care of constipation and heartburn, and that osteoporosis (like other major health problems) cannot be prevented with some supplements but only with a healthy, natural diet? No, they would not tell you because they are smart.

In this world not the strong anymore but only the smart survive. Be smarter than them when you walk into a supermarket. Get smart; do not turn your home into a junk food restaurant. Your life and your children's life and future depend on it!

In all fairness, we have to admit that we cannot put all the blame on the junk food makers; cigarettes and booze are made, advertised, and sold everywhere, and yet, not everyone is an alcoholic and/or a smoker.

You as a potential consumer are the subject of a plot. Smart people want to make money on you. That would be okay if they gave you a great service and cared about your health; but they do not! So you have to be smarter than them. None of those who get rich on you will be there to help you when you get colon cancer, breast cancer, or a heart attack from their cheap, greasy, over-processed food, or when your child becomes a diabetic from all the sugar our food is laced with. Probably, the same people will sell the child insulin just to make him reach the time when his legs have to be amputated. (Sorry, when you know the facts, it is hard not to get carried away, not to get emotionally involved.)

It is a jungle out there. It is a fight for your health and life every day. Of course, at first glance it sounds like a gross exaggeration, but every time you walk through the door of a restaurant or a supermarket, the chances are that you take a step closer to cancer, heart attacks, diabetes, osteoporoses, etc. Those small steps add up.

The food manufacturer looks at the consumer the way the farmer looks at his pig: let us feed him the cheapest stuff, so that we can make the highest profit. It is hard to believe, right? Just look at the labels on cookies: most are made with coconut oil, the manufacturers' favorite, because it is cheap. It is cheap, because it is of very low quality. In fact, it is so bad that the coconut-growing natives used to make soap of it; now we are buying it for our kids. (Most non-dairy cream substitutes are made of this "raw soap", which is a lot worse than the cholesterol in cream!)

By New Year's Eve every year, about one million of us die terrible deaths needlessly, in addition to the countless others who suffer discomfort or disability, as the direct result of disease-promoting life-styles.

To say the least, it is very hard to find healthy food. We hope that what you read in this guide will help you identify harmful, neutral, and beneficial substances. What you take home from the supermarket is extremely important, since that is what you and your family will eat and drink the following day(s).

Our mass-produced meat is polluted with about 150 different kinds of growth-stimulating hormones, tranquilizers, antibiotics, herbicides, fungicides, and pesticides. In addition to all these, bacterial and viral infections are so common that they are almost considered "normal". High- ranking government officials publicly admit, for instance, that 35 - 50% of the chickens in supermarkets are infected with salmonella, and people are dying from it. Hundreds of millions of animals are discarded every year because of cancer and birth defects caused by what is added to their feed and drinking water or injected into them. *"Naturally"*, *those carcasses are utilized as feed for other animals.*

About 2000 different kinds of drugs and chemicals are mixed regularly with animal feed. Artificial colors are added to give "natural" color to the skin or the eggyolk; arsenic is added to accelerate growth and egg production; preservatives are added to prevent spoilage of fish ground up for feed, etc.

Many of the additives are suspected to be carcinogenic or mutagenic, and have never been thoroughly tested. Hundreds of millions of tons of chemicals are used annualy in the agriculture of the U.S.; dozens of them leave residues in the crops. *The residues are most likely to accumulate in fat,* which gives us one more reason to stay away from meat and limit the consumption of eggs, sour cream, milk, and butter. Probably, deep-sea fish are the best choice of all the animals when it comes to healthy foods.

Health inspectors openly admit that there is no time for thorough checking; they have about 3 seconds(!) per animal. Moreover, by the time the test results are known, the meat product is already long gone from the supermarket shelf.

In excess, even natural meat is harmful, but try to imagine our mass-produced, "manufactured" meats. Perhaps, you would never touch a hotdog again if you saw the "raw material" before the chemicals are added to make it red (instead of grey), and to make it taste like meat (instead of sawdust).

THE "AVOID!" LIST

1. *Bacon, meat* - in any form: raw, cooked, canned, smoked, grilled or barbecued, such as sausage, salami, frankfurter, or ham.

Meat is about 50% fat in terms of caloric value; all processed meat products contain harmful chemical preservatives. Do not think you have to have meat every day; your body would like to have it (or rather tolerate it) only once a week. By avoiding meat, you will take a big step toward preventing heart attack, blood vessel diseases, breast cancer, colon cancer and cancers at other sites, osteoporosis, obesity, hemorrhoids, constipation, and everything else that all the hormone, tranquilizer, herbicide, antibiotics, pesticide and fungicide residues and the preservatives can cause. Simply, take meat home only on rare occasions. Treat yourself to a meat meal once or twice a week; enjoy it; make it a special treat.

2. *Refined sugar, corn syrup* - in any form: candies, cookies, ice cream, pastries, cakes, canned fruits in syrup, cake mixes and everything else laced with sugar.

Always read the label. Simply, take home nothing that has sugar in it. Diabetes, obesity, vitamin and mineral deficiencies, cancer, elevated blood cholesterol level, heart disease, and cavities can be the result of the "shock treatment" your organs receive from sugary products.

3. *White flour, white rice* - in any form: most commercial baked goods, cake mixes, stuffings, breads, muffins, breakfast cereals, pastas, noodles, crackers, cookies, white rice, and "quick" rice.

If the label says 'enriched' or 'unbleached ', even if it is colored brown, it is still just cheap white flour. Over-processed cereal products go hand in hand with fatty and sugary foods in causing all the "modern" diseases mentioned previously.

We cannot overemphasize the importance of fiber. It is literally a matter of life and death. Thousands upon thousands of food products of plant origin line the shelves in an average foodstore, but over 90% of them have almost no fiber left in them after the "manufacturing" process. To find the right stuff, you have to be a sleuth; there is a jungle out there.

4. *All soft drinks* - even if it is "diet".

They contain sugar or corn syrup or their chemical substitutes with other potentially dangerous chemicals (some of them are simply called "artificial colors and artificial flavors"). Most soft drinks are a murky brew of chemicals undrinkable at room temperature. *The universally despised tapwater is a smarter bet if cooled and diluted with some fruit juice.*

Due to excessive amounts of phosphoric acid in almost all soft drinks - beside diabetes, heart damage, cancer and many other health hazards - osteoporosis is threatening primarily women and children with smaller skeletons and lesser overall body-weight. As a result of many factors (among them very intensive advertising), soft drink consumption is increasing at a rate never seen before. The long-term effect of this new phenomenon, coupled with a similar dependence on sugary, salty, fatty, fiber-free, deficient junk food, is impossible to foresee.

5. *Fruit juices* - unless you mix them with 9 parts of water to 1 part juice.

Even if not laced with refined sugar or corn syrup, fruit juices can disturb blood sugar level regulation. Most of them have very little fiber, and might create a craving for other sweet drinks and foods.

Your body was not meant to handle what you guzzle as water substitute. It even has to draw water from the blood to the intestines to handle the sugar, salt and other substances in the juice which was supposedly introduced to dilute bodily fluids, but became the subject of digestive processes, since it is thicker than the fluids in your system. So, it is obvious: clear water is the best thirst-quencher. *There is no substitute for the real thing!*

6. *Miscellaneous*

Vegetable oils sold in supermarkets have nothing left of their original nutritional value. Most of them are solvent extracted (using benzine or hexane) or pressed at high temperatures, then "processed" into a substance that has very little to do with Nature. Even BHT (a carcinogenic) is added to preserve "quality".

If these "oils" are hydrogenated, they completely lose touch with Nature. Do not even touch them. At high temperature, vegetable oils become carcinogenic. Never use them for frying; saute instead in butter or peanut oil or virgin olive oil.

Avoid mayonnaise, salad dressing, sandwich spread, sweetened and colored yogurt, pastry, canned food, meat products, and "T.V. dinners" that contain artificial flavor and artificial color, preservatives, coconut or palm oil, or hydrogenated oil (even if it's "partially").

Avoid convenience snack foods, such as, potato chips, cheese-puffs, and coated popcorn. Find sensible alternatives (fruits, nuts, seeds, etc.)

As for cigarettes, alcohol, and coffee, do not buy them! Many millions live without them, or stopped abusing them; you can, too!

ONLY YOU CAN DO IT!

"Man-made", over-processed foods have a shocking effect every time you eat them. Well-orchestrated processes, practiced for billions of years, are disrupted. *Your system simply does not know how to relate to sudden energy rushes, little bulk, or "never-seen" chemicals.*

Organs and cells start acting "funny" after a while; they produce too much or not enough of certain substances; they move things too fast or too slow. In this chaos, those strange chemicals are doing their destructive work unchecked. Names have been invented for these conditions: diabetes (too little insulin); hypoglycemia (too much insulin), cancer (too many cells reproduced too fast); atherosclerosis (too much fat deposited and too fast in the blood vessels); constipation, colon cancer, appendicitis, diverticulitis, ulcers (little bulk, the "surprised" intestines move it slowly, allowing some substances to cause damage). This goes on and on like a chain reaction.

Osteoporosis is probably caused by the lack of calcium, but most probably by excess phosphorus from meat, soft drinks and many other deficient foods. Nobody really knows how it works exactly, but nobody is looking for a virus or a bacterium, as nobody is looking for the "germ" that causes diabetes or heart attacks either. We have already defeated almost all the germs that cause life-threatening diseases. Doctors have a relatively easy job with germs: they just have to kill those creatures, and everything is all right. The victims of the new plagues of civilization are not helped by simple hypodermic injections.

Yes, indeed, most of these diseases are **incurable**. Never forget that! But some of them are **reversible**. Never forget that either! And never, never forget that **THEY ARE PREVENTABLE** ! Anytime you go into a restaurant or buy food and drink for yourself and your loved ones, be aware of this. Also, be aware of the fact that a smart person is able to get the same amount of satisfaction out of good food as junk food.

Learn to care about your health. Nobody else will do it for you.
Only you can do it!

NOW, WHAT?

Most of us are told from time to time to cut back on this or to cut back on that. If we cut back on everything we eat, what are we going to eat? This guide is also special in the sense that it tells you what to substitute for "normal" - that is, junk food - without confining you to a strict regimen.

Eating is a joy, but it is a headache, as well, at least three times a day. If you have a family, you can multiply that with the number of the family members.

Laziness is as ancient as greed and many other "noble" traits of man, so most of us prefer foods that are convenient. In this sense, convenience is measured by the time it takes to prepare something before we gobble it up - regardless of its contents. The problem is that the "ready-to-eat" foods are not "prepared" but manufactured and preserved by chemicals in order to last; in other words: they are bad for you.

Other than knowledge, we think, laziness and poverty are the two major factors that can greatly contribute to your health. The ever-present laziness is no problem. Lack of poverty might cause some difficulties; nowhere else on the earth is food as cheap as here in the U.S. In other countries people think ten times before they buy meat or go to a restaurant ; we might think twice. The only thing we have to do is to pretend that we are poor. It is not a joke; it is dead serious.

A great deal depends on what you buy in the stores and restaurants. Do not buy the products of the Avoid! List. It seems you save all the money you normally spend on food, right? But it is not the case; there are some healthy foods around. If you get only the healthy stuff, you save about 30% on the monthly food budget.

Of course, you will be tempted to buy occasionally some "Avoid" items; but do not keep them at home in the refrigerator or anywhere else. This way you will not be exposed to temptations while at home. If you wish to sin, you will have to go to the market first; and here comes in laziness.

Now comes pretending poverty. It is harder than you think. Processed foods are far more expensive than their raw form, still, we buy them. We tend to look down on unprocessed foods, as sort of "poor man's diet". Have you ever seen lentils advertised? Many people do not even know what lentils are. There is not too much profit in it, so you will never see it on television. It is "just" one of the most nutritious foods money can buy. Using lentils you can prepare a meal for a family of six(!), at a cost of about two dollars and thirty minutes. For the same number of people, a pizza will cost about twelve dollars - and their health. You be the judge as to which way is smarter.

So be smart, and find the best foods in the labyrinth of the supermarkets. Here is a list of them:

1. **Fruits & Nuts & Seeds** - apples, peaches, apricots, cherries, plums, strawberries, oranges, blueberries, grapefruit, watermelon, cantaloupe, pears, bananas, grapes, tangerines etc. Almonds, peanuts, pistachios, walnuts, cashews, sunflower seeds, pecans, water chestnuts.

Make it a habit to keep plenty at home all the time. When you have got the "munchies", substitute fruits for pastries, ice cream or potato chips. Remember, the long-living in Vilcabamba and Hunza almost literally live on fruits. You cannot eat too much of them. You will not gain weight, since they contain mainly water and fiber. You have to be a bit careful only with avocados, seeds and nuts.

2. **Vegetables** - carrots, parsley (roots and leaves), green peas, green beans, spinach, kohlrabi, turnips, rutabagas, raddish, lettuce, celery, cucumber, cauliflower, Brussel sprouts, broccoli, collards, potatoes, onions, lettuce, sweet potatoes, corn, bell peppers, kale, tomatoes, cabbage, etc.

Make it a habit to keep plenty at home. When you have got the "munchies", eat raw carrots, or kohlrabi, or celery, or a whole-grain bread sandwich with a thin slice of light cheese and lots of tomato, bell pepper, raddish, etc. on it. You just cannot eat too much of a sandwich like that, you do not have to worry about gaining weight.

It makes no sense at all to buy canned or "bagged" soups. Manufactured instant soups have less nutritional value and fiber, and usually are laced with salt and chemicals. It takes just a little effort to prepare a healthy meal enough for the whole family for a day or two.

Do not worry if the fruits or vegetables are not fresh. We are one of the few nations where almost everything is available all the time, regardless of the seasons. Others, among them the long-living, have to settle for preserved food during the winter and early spring.

3. **Dry legumes** - beans, peas, lentils, soybean.

Here comes again the problem of poverty. Legumes and potatoes are considered the poor man's diet, and indeed they are almost free in this country (if unprocessed). Nevertheless, legumes are extremely healthy, rich in protein, vitamins, minerals and fiber, and sustain almost the entire population of the world.

This is part of the "secret" of the centenarians; legumes, potatoes, whole grain breads, supplemented with vegetables, fruits and nuts, fermented dairy products, and occasionally some meat, *give them the healthiest, best-balanced regimen this world has to offer.*

So, do not feel deprived if there is no sausage on your plate every morning, or if days go by without meat, fried potatoes, or pastry. *The poor man's diet is the smart man's diet.*

4. **Grain Crops** - wheat, barley, millet, rice, rye, oats, triticale, corn, buckwheat, bulgur, amaranth.

It is of vital importance that you always have around breads, cookies, tortillas, crackers, pretzels, and other baked goods *made only with whole-grain flour.* Avoid anything with a label that says "enriched", "unbleached" or simply states "wheat flour". Never buy white rice; instead, get only brown (short or long grain).

5. **Miscellaneous**

Spices - red pepper, black pepper, thyme, salt, celery seeds, bay leaves, sweet basil, coriander, cumin, rosemary, garlic, mayonnaise, mustard, horseradish, oregano, caraway seeds, all-natural salt-free mix of spices, etc.

Fats and *oils* - lard, butter, cold-pressed virgin olive oil, peanut oil, and cottonseed oil.

Lard and butter definitely sound like an "off-the-wall" suggestion in the light of decades of indoctrination to force us to use "healthy" vegetable oils and margarine. Because of the hurried mass-production, the vegetable oil industry turns out worthless and harmful "lubricant", which turns carcinogenic when heated. The wisdom of Nature shines again in providing people with something that is not that harmful. Indeed, instead of vegetable oils, lard (tallow in the Caucasus and Hunza), butter and cold-pressed walnut oil have been used by the centenarians. But the real key to the problem is quantity: they always use just a bit on the tip of a spoon.

Never deep-fry anything. If you dislike lard and butter, keep at home *only a small bottle* of virgin olive oil, or peanut oil, or cottonseed oil (all monounsaturated); always use a small amount only. Try to saute (in butter or oil) instead of frying.

Dairy products - plain yogurt, kefir, cottage or farmer's cheese, low-fat cheeses, feta cheese.

Never run out of these foods; they are incomparably more valuable than the meat products which many in this country consider indispensable to our breakfast, lunch, dinner, and every sandwich. (*Stay away from sour cream*: *it is almost pure fat*.)

6. Water

Having the clearest water possible in your home all the time, should be at the top of your list of priorities. The foods listed above require more water than modern junk food in order to be digested in the intestines and to pass through your system smoothly. In light of the widespread pollution, it is of utmost importance for everybody to have *bottled mountain spring water* available any time, or to have a water cleaning system with *carbon blocks* as filtering agent. Use only clean water for drinking and cooking. *The tap water is far more contaminated than you might think.*

When drinking a soft drink, think of the "possibility" that the manufacturers do not go out of their way to make the water cleaner than tap water before they mix it with their brew. We customers pay 36 billion dollars a year for their "services". It is truly incredible! The money you save by ignoring sodas, will buy for you the best water cleaning system - and, perhaps, a cruise to the Caribbean.

MAKE IT A HABIT!

It takes time to pick up bad habits, and it takes time (and effort, of course) to get rid of them. It also takes time to pick up, again, good habits. By constantly practicing good things, soon you will have good habits naturally replacing the old bad ones. So keep practicing, start right away!

Make it a habit not to smoke.
Make it a habit to have no more than two alcoholic drinks a day, if any.
Make it a habit to drink clear water and eat several times a day.
Make it a habit to eat and drink small amounts each time.
Make it a habit to bag yourself a lunch if there is no other way to eat healthy food at work (plus you will save a lot of money, too).
Make it a habit to buy no food or drink if it has chemical preservatives, sugar, white flour, artificial sweetener, flavor, or color, hydrogenated, coconut or palm oil in it, or if it is smoked or deep-fried.
Make it a habit not to keep "Avoid!" items at home. (This way, if you yield to temptation, you have to go and get them.)

This last sentence "takes care" of 90 to 95% of the foods sold in supermarkets. The Laws of Profit dictate that food manufacturers should use cheap raw material and make it last. The foods in most of those shiny boxes, bags, jars, or cans meet this requirement but not that of the common sense.

As customer awareness is increasing, more and more healthy products appear on the market. Now you can get even in the supermarkets whole grain spaghetti, preservative-free salad dressing, mustard, tuna, and bread, sugar-free peanut butter, jam, and fruit juices.

But we are not "aware" enough, so giant manufacturers are not forced yet to make only good food for us. Without a second thought of promoting anyone's business, we have to recommend for you to discover the health food stores and the farmers markets in your area. *Vote with your money for healthy food.* Shop frequently at these places where you can get unsprayed and organic grains, fruits, and vegetables; whole-grain cookies, breads, spaghetti, and pasta; sugarless ice cream; healthy sandwiches, salads, light cheeses, unsalted butter, plain kefir and yogurt, cold-pressed vegetable oils; chemical-free salad dressing, natural breakfast cereals, etc. *This is as close as you can get to natural foods these days -* unless you have a farm.

More and more people are getting all the food they need from health food stores and farmers markets. Prices normally are higher than in supermarkets, but it is still more economical, because if one eats unprocessed foods, eats less due to their wholesomeness. Compare a piece of fat-soaked hamburger between two papery buns and a whole-grain sandwich. The whole-grain is simply more filling - makes you feel full longer - and richer in vitamins, fiber, minerals and vital fatty acids.

All in all, consumers of unprocessed foods save money - and their good health.

The more people turn towards alternative sources, the more attention supermarkets will have to pay to ordering healthy foodstuffs. We are seeing a rapid increase in the number of farmers who cultivate their crops without artificial fertilizers and herbicides. It takes some thinking and planning ahead, rotating and combining certain plants, but it is possible. The real good news is that the non-chemical way is more productive: 50 % more corn can be produced at one-fifth of the cost of chemical farming. Healthier, more productive, protects the environment - let us vote for it with our purchases.

It is an unmatchable feeling to know that you are eating the healthiest food available. You will feel strong, light, healthy, and confident. You will feel good about yourself all over.

It takes some time to pick up a habit, so make it a habit to practice what you have learned from this guide. No matter how long the journey is; every step counts. Even the smallest change for the better counts. And it is far easier than you think.

PHYSICAL ACTIVITY

The limited space devoted to this topic is not an indication that exercise is not important. There has been so much fuss about it (just like about "diets"), that many feel guilty if a day goes by without a thorough "work-out".

Our approach is very simple in this case, too. The centenarians are never doing fancy exercises; the same simple rhythmical movements: walking, leaning forward many times a day, lifting lighter things, day after day, are the other major contributors (along with their natural diet) to their exceptional physical fitness.

The long-living are never running or jogging, so just make it simple: walk, swim, row. Of course, light running or jogging also can be beneficial with adequate preparation. Our point is: do not expect better results from running or aerobic dance classes than from walking just because they are more exhausting. *Instead of trying exercises that demand oxygen and energy, your muscles (among them the heart) need slower, sustained rhythmical movements that help build up the supply lines of oxygen and energy.*

Indeed, it is a scientifically proven fact that **walking makes the heart and the blood vessels stronger than aerobic exercise.**

It is so sad to see many (most of them elderly) running in city parks and streets, who do not even know how to run. For the unprepared, running can be dangerous. It is just like someone trying to build strengh and large muscles by lifting the heaviest weights that he can; injury, pain and disappointment can be the result. Walking, swimming or rowing are the "light weights" that give your muscles and organs time to slowly adapt and develop, building up long-lasting benefits.

Consider the obvious: if you run up 200 steps you might even die, but walking the same steps two or three times daily will build for you a really strong heart.

Few athletes live long, so do not overstrain yourself. But, do not live a sedentary life-style either. Instead, make it a habit to walk, swim or row about 20 - 30 minutes 3 times a week at least - but at least on the weekends.

Regular exercise relieves stress, promotes strong bones and muscles, even makes the skin smoother, shinier.

Walking is the most ancient "exercise", and the safest. Walking is like fruits: you cannot have too much of it. Still, you are cautioned to start a new exercise program always gradually.

For the days when you do not have a chance to walk outside, a rowing machine comes handy. Considering the large number of muscles it moves, rowing is perhaps the second best exercise (after walking).

A study of the life-style of 17,000 people, male graduates of a major university (Harvard), has revealed that the death rate was approximately 50 % lower among those who exercised regularly. *The life of the active ones was prolonged by as much as 20 %*; that is about 10 - 15 years of quality time. Think about it.

Of course, it is not just a matter of exercise: it is a prudent assumption to say, that who is health-conscious enough to exercise regularly, is health-conscious enough to choose healthy food over junk food.

STRESS

The daily life of the centenarians are not free of problems, but undoubtedly less stressful than ours. Most of them very seldom leave the place at which they grew up. No significant changes take place in their diet or the way they eat, work, and live in general. On the other hand, the "civilized man" is exposed to constantly changing factors and uncertainty both inside and outside the family circles.

The "pill" against stress is yet to be discovered. It is probably as hopeless as trying to find the "virus" that causes heart attacks.

Probably, the best way to cope with stress is to be infinitely patient and understanding with each other. This applies to spouses, neighbors, fellow workers, etc. Most of us are not that way, but like many other skills, it can be learned. Listening to what the other has to say, talking everything over slowly and quietly is a far better way to deal with problems. Yelling at each other solves nothing but creates more tension.

Some physical activity (walking, gardening, going to the movies, etc.) is also very effective - especially if it is done together with someone. **During physical activity, the body produces morphine-like substances: endorphines. That is why we feel good after a reasonable amount of physical exertion.**

Try not to get upset over anything which you have no control over anyway (like traffic jams, or the "stupidity" of someone else). When sitting in the middle of a traffic jam, try to feel satisfied that at least there is time to think some important things over. Never get mad at anybody; just try to ignore the other person, who might have a very good reason to act the way he is acting. Or perhaps, the other party *is* what you think he is: stupid. That is not a blessing. *Feel sorry for him, instead.*

If nothing helps, try to think how insignificant the situation you are in will be 100 years later.

We believe our simple approach to stress control is as effective as anything else. *Make it a habit to practice it.* You will see that this is the only way to do it.

CHILDREN

This guide has been intended to help children more than anybody else. Millions of them are the victims of lust, greed, indifference and ignorance of adults. It is a sad fact that *millions of innocent little people are victimized right in front of our eyes: they are offered, or rather forced to live on a regimen that has claimed millions of lives, and caused inexplicable misery to millions more.*

Armies of well-trained and well-paid professionals are doing their best to entice children to consume more and more of their "products".

Due to their undeveloped bodies, lower body weight, and weeker immune system, children are more vulnerable than adults. Many are exposed to hundreds of chemicals, hormones, tranquilizers, alcohol, caffeine, smoke, smog, drugs, sugar, etc. - even before birth !

We adults have to give them a helping hand, instead. Pregnant mothers have to stay away from anything unnatural. Eat and drink only natural things - and God or Nature will take care of the rest for you. Babies need to be fed (preferably breastfed) mother's milk as long as possible, and mashed peas, lentils, potato, fruits, spinach, etc. as soon as possible. (The centenarians started eating these when they were 6 months old or even younger.)

Their lunch menu needs to be checked. Most schools cannot offer better food than a junk food restaurant. A whole-grain sandwich with some fruit is healthier than some "scientifically designed" lunches.

Quite understandably, children show great resistance towards changing the diet they are used to, but according to our experiments, they can be convinced with relative ease. When thoroughly explained, even the very young will enthusiastically agree with and support a shift toward a healthier regimen. *They will be even proud of themselves*: they will feel that they are smarter than other kids and adults who do not know how to care for themselves. They will feel sorry for people buying chemical-laden drinks and chemical-laden, over-processed foods in restaurants and grocery stores.

If once a week you still let them "sin", a slice of pizza or a hamburger will taste like something from the heaven, and the trip to the restaurant will be a special treat.

Limit their time in front of the television. Create some interest in them for reading; help them in the beginning to aquire the basic math skills. From then on, they will be on their way to learn everything they can. They will view the world more openmindedly; will feel confident and good about themselves. This is for a sound mind.

For a sound body, beside teaching them a healthy diet, let them play (but not video games, for God's sake); *take them with you on walkings, hikings, swimmings, etc. Encourage physical activity any way you can.*

Schools cannot be relied on in this case. To the best of our knowledge, the U.S. stands alone among the developed nations as the one without extensive physical education program in schools (with the exception of Illinois and a few other states).

By the time high school graduation comes, the average U.S. student will have spent about 15,000 hours in front of the television set, as opposed to 13,000 hours of school education. And there is very little good one can learn from the TV programs after reaching the age of 10.

Forty percent(!) *of our children between 6 and 12 years of age already show symptoms that clearly lead to heart attack.* **No generation ever before had such a bad start. Who could foresee the long-term effects?**

THIS IS THE ONLY WAY TO DO IT!

Every system is maintained through the delicate balances between its components. When exterior or interior forces disrupt the balance, some kind of change will take place. If the balance disrupted was a kind we wanted to maimtain, we call the change deterioration. Like all living things, the human body is constantly deteriorating (or aging). Despite this little understood, "built-in" self-distruction program, human beings can live longer than many other creatures.

What we breathe or swallow becomes instantly part of our system, so obviously, **your diet or life-style in general can promote balance or disruption, thus, you have control over slowing down or accelerating the aging process.** With their long life the centenarians have shown the world that their diet and life-style are the closest to perfect.

"Miracle formulas" and other ointments will not make you stay young; **only a diet and life-style close to those of the centenarians can prevent premature aging.** If you follow them as much as you can, you will do everything in your power. Your hair will stay dark longer; your skin will stay smooth and shiny longer; you will feel young longer - indeed, you will be young longer.

There are many things you have no control over, but with knowledge and constantly increasing awareness, you can easily widen the sphere of influence over your destiny. Be always aware of your possibilities and the responsibilities for your own health and that of others.

Make it a habit to practice what you have learned from this guide. **Make it part of your life.** Knowledge is power; power is freedom. With this knowledge you will achieve in your personal life two of the greatest feelings: health and freedom.

Only you can do it, and this is the only way to do it!

THE "SMART MAN'S DIET"

Here you find no real recipes but a few simple ideas for how to make healthy meals quickly. *We are convinced that the know-how of a few simple concoctions, which you can make with little effort and time, is worth more than a whole library of cookbooks.* Exotic recipes from exotic cookbooks are purposely not included in the guide, because cookbooks, by their very nature, always contain the fanciest recipes not the simple meals people actually live on.

We recommend that you rely on a short list you can compile by adding your favorite recipes to our ideas. In any library, hundreds of cookbooks offer inexhaustible sources of recipes. You just have to find the right ones for you. And now you know what is good for you. The most important thing is: **make it simple**.

If you live on a healthy diet, it will not really matter if you eat some "undesirable" meals every once in a while. A great deal depends on what is kept in the kitchen and whether you are willing to put a little effort into preparing healthy meals for yourself. Nobody will do it for you.

Here is a list of what should be thrown out immediately and should not be bought and stored in your kitchen:

(This is a short form of the "Avoid!" list)

Meat - fresh, frozen, cured, smoked, processed in any way
White flour - or anything made with it
White rice - in any form and shape
Sugar - white or brown, and anything made with it
Sour cream, fatty, smoked cheeses
Vegetable oil - *unless it is certified "cold-pressed"*
Anything that has artificial flavors or colors, preservatives,
palm oil, coconut oil, hydrogenated vegetable oil
Anything deep-fried - chicken, potato chips, etc.

Soft drinks - any kind
Alcohol
Cigarettes
Drugs

Shopping List

Whole grains - brown rice, oats, whole-grain flour, bread, tortilla, pastas, bagels, muffins, shreded wheat cereal, etc.
Legumes - dry beans, peas, lentils
Vegetables - whatever you can think of, including potatoes, onions, string beans, even garlic
Fruits - whatever you can think of
Nuts - whatever you can think of
Yogurt - plain only
Farmer's or cottage cheese
Kefir
Milk - do not buy it by the gallon, and do not use it as substitute for water
Cheese - white and light, use it sparingly
Butter - unsalted, use it sparingly
Honey - uncooked, unfiltered, use it sparingly
Oil - cold-pressed virgin olive or peanut oil; use it sparingly
Eggs - use them sparingly
Spices
Clear water
Add here what you like and still healthy (e.g. sardines, tuna, popcorn, etc.)

If you keep these items at home, the more you eat at home the healthier you will be. Eat your breakfast at home as often as you can. Make quickly 1 or 2 sandwiches for lunch; always pack some fruits, also. The chances are that you will find only junk food when you are away from your home.

Nowhere else in the world is cooking as easy as in the U.S. Cook something simple as often as you can get yourself to do it. Make enough for 2 days. Use the leftovers the next day. Do not feel denied: this "poor man's diet" is the diet of the smart.

Here are a few simple ideas. Follow the footsteps of the centenarians: make it simple.

Almond bean sprouts   (*this half is for your ideas*)

½ cup almonds (sliced)
3 cup bean sprouts
½ cup bell pepper
½ cup carrot (grated)
½ cup celery (diced)
½ cup green onion (chopped)
Dressing:
2 tbsp mayonnaise
2 tbsp soy sause
dash of curry and ginger

Can be "enriched" with parmesan, mozzarella, or feta cheese.
Ingredients can be substituted with your favorites or whatever found in your refrigerator.

Broccoli pasta

3 cup pasta (cooked)
1 cup broccoli (small pieces)
½ cup olives
2   green onion (chopped)
½ cup goat or feta cheese (crumbled)
3 tbsp olive oil
2 tbsp vinegar
dash of salt and black pepper

Macaroni green pea salad

3 cup elbow macaroni (cooked)
½ cup celery (diced)
1 cup green peas (boiled 1 min.)
½ cup tomato (sliced)
½ bnch parsley leaves (chopped)
2 clve garlic (minced)
2   green onion (chopped)
½ cup mayonnaise
1 tbsp mustard
2 tbsp vinegar
black pepper and salt to taste

Rice salad

3 cup rice (cooked slowly 30-45
     minutes in 5 cups of water)
½ cup nuts of your choice (sliced)
½ cup celery (diced)
½ cup olives
¼ cup parsley leaves (chopped)
½ cup bell pepper (diced)
3   green onion (chopped)
2 clve garlic (minced)
1 tbsp red wine vinegar
1 tbsp mustard
1 tesp oregano
1 tesp basil
1 tesp tarragon

To make it even simpler, add only the green onion (sauteed in 2 tbsp oil),
3 eggs, and soy sauce to the rice.

Barley salad

3 cup barley (cooked slowly 1.5 hr.
     in 5 cups of water)
2 cup broccoli (sauteed or raw)
1 cup carrot (diced, sauteed or raw)
½ cup green onion (chopped)
½ cup red/green bell pepper (diced)
½ cup nuts of your choice (sliced)
2 clve garlic (minced)
½ cup lemon juice
5 tbsp olive oil
1 tesp sweet basil
dash of thyme, salt, black/red pepper

Yogurt dressing

1 cup yogurt
½ cup buttermilk
2 tbsp parsley leaves (minced)
½ tbsp curry powder
1 tesp honey
salt or pepper to taste
2 clve garlic (minced, optional)

Yogurt with fruit

1 cup yogurt
1 tesp honey

Add diced fruits of your choice. Cottage cheese can be substituted for or mixed with yogurt.

Sandwiches

Use little butter, or thin slice of cheese, or breadspread; eat lots of bell pepper, tomato, etc. with it.

Liptói breadspread

½ cup feta cheese (crumbled)
¼ cup yogurt
1 tbsp butter
2 tbsp green onion (chopped)
1 tesp ground caraway seed
dash of salt and sweet paprika

Vegetable bean stew

2 cup beans (of your choice)
5 qt. water
1 cup each: onion, parsley roots,
     turnip (or of your preference)
4 clve garlic
salt, black pepper, paprika
1 cup yogurt (optional)

Cook beans 1.5 hr., then add vegetables for another 15 minutes. Add yogurt to pot or individual bowls.

Lentil stew

2 cup lentils
6 cup water
1 cup onion (chopped)
1 cup yogurt
4   bay leaves
4 clve garlic (minced)
4 tbsp olive oil
2 tbsp wheat flour
salt and paprika to taste

Cook lentils with bay leaves for 30 min., while you saute onion; then mix flour with onion, after 1 min. add garlic, spices, and yogurt, then add this gravy to lentils. Dilute stew with milk (opt.). Eat it with whole-grain bread.

Split pea soup

3 cup dry peas
6 cup water
1 cup carrot (diced)
½ cup celery (diced)
½ cup turnip (diced)
½ cup onion (diced)
3 clve garlic (minced)
dash of oregano and thyme; black pepper, salt, paprika to taste

Cook peas 45 min., then add spices and vegetables for 15 min. If you prefer, blend it in mixer. Eat it with whole-grain bread.

Stuffed potato

8   large potato
1 cup cheddar cheese (grated)
½ cup yogurt
1 tbsp butter
2 tesp paprika
1 tesp black pepper
½ bnch green onion (chopped)
salt to taste.

Bake potatoes about 1 hr. at 350 degr., then cut them in half, cut out the inside part, mix it with ingredients, but put cheese on top; bake them for 10 min.
To save time, use microwave oven; taste will be different.

Pancake

Adding more milk to your regular pancake batter will make the pancakes thinner, so that they could be rolled and stuffed with apple sauce or cottage cheese mixed with little honey. Do not use butter or syrup.

2   egg
1¼ cup whole-wheat flour
1 cup milk
1 cup carbonated water

Spinach balls

3 cup frozen spinach (thaw it, sqeeze
          juice out)
1 cup cheddar cheese (grated)
1   egg
bread crumbs, salt, black pepper as needed
chopped onion and garlic optional

Mix ingredients, shape balls, bake them 10 min. at 350 degr. (Hamburger can be shaped as well.)

AWARENESS CALENDAR

Filling out this calendar at the end of each week for a while, will help you monitor your progress as you are picking up "long-life" habits.

Week #__ Date:_____
I had

fresh or cooked vegetables		__days
fresh fruits		__days
100 % whole grain		__days
cooked dry legumes		__days
nuts and seeds		__days
plain fermented dairy products		__days
I walked	__min/mi	__days
swam	__min/yd	__days
rowed	__min	__days
jogged	__min/mi	__days
did aerobics	__min	__days
_____	_____	__days

Week #__ Date:_____
I had

fresh or cooked vegetables		__days
fresh fruits		__days
100 % whole grain		__days
cooked dry legumes		__days
nuts and seeds		__days
plain fermented dairy products		__days
I walked	__min/mi	__days
swam	__min/yd	__days
rowed	__min	__days
jogged	__min/mi	__days
did aerobics	__min	__days
_____	_____	__days

Week #__ Date:_____
I had
fresh or cooked vegetables   __days
fresh fruits   __days
100 % whole grain   __days
cooked dry legumes   __days
nuts and seeds   __days
plain fermented dairy products   __days
I walked   __min/mi   __days
 swam   __min/yd   __days
 rowed   __min   __days
 jogged   __min/mi   __days
 did aerobics   __min   __days
 _____   _____   __days

Week #__ Date:_____
I had
fresh or cooked vegetables   __days
fresh fruits   __days
100 % whole grain   __days
cooked dry legumes   __days
nuts and seeds   __days
plain fermented dairy products   __days
I walked   __min/mi   __days
 swam   __min/yd   __days
 rowed   __min   __days
 jogged   __min/mi   __days
 did aerobics   __min   __days
 _____   _____   __days

Week #__ Date:_____
I had
fresh or cooked vegetables   __days
fresh fruits   __days
100 % whole grain   __days
cooked dry legumes   __days
nuts and seeds   __days
plain fermented dairy products   __days
I walked   __min/mi   __days
   swam   __min/yd   __days
   rowed   __min   __days
   jogged   __min/mi   __days
   did aerobics   __min   __days
  _____   _____   __days

Week #__ Date:_____
I had
fresh or cooked vegetables   __days
fresh fruits   __days
100 % whole grain   __days
cooked dry legumes   __days
nuts and seeds   __days
plain fermented dairy products   __days
I walked   __min/mi   __days
   swam   __min/yd   __days
   rowed   __min   __days
   jogged   __min/mi   __days
   did aerobics   __min   __days
  _____   _____   __days

Week #__ Date:_____
I had
fresh or cooked vegetables   __days
fresh fruits   __days
100 % whole grain   __days
cooked dry legumes   __days
nuts and seeds   __days
plain fermented dairy products   __days
I walked   __min/mi   __days
  swam   __min/yd   __days
  rowed   __min   __days
  jogged   __min/mi   __days
  did aerobics   __min   __days
_____   _____   __days

Week #__ Date:_____
I had
fresh or cooked vegetables   __days
fresh fruits   __days
100 % whole grain   __days
cooked dry legumes   __days
nuts and seeds   __days
plain fermented dairy products   __days
I walked   __min/mi   __days
  swam   __min/yd   __days
  rowed   __min   __days
  jogged   __min/mi   __days
  did aerobics   __min   __days
_____   _____   __days

Week #__ Date:_____
I had
fresh or cooked vegetables   __days
fresh fruits   __days
100 % whole grain   __days
cooked dry legumes   __days
nuts and seeds   __days
plain fermented dairy products   __days
I walked   __min/mi   __days
  swam   __min/yd   __days
  rowed   __min   __days
  jogged   __min/mi   __days
  did aerobics   __min   __days
_____   _____   __days

Week #__ Date:_____
I had
fresh or cooked vegetables   __days
fresh fruits   __days
100 % whole grain   __days
cooked dry legumes   __days
nuts and seeds   __days
plain fermented dairy products   __days
I walked   __min/mi   __days
  swam   __min/yd   __days
  rowed   __min   __days
  jogged   __min/mi   __days
  did aerobics   __min   __days
_____   _____   __days

Week #__ Date:_____
I had
fresh or cooked vegetables   __days
fresh fruits   __days
100 % whole grain   __days
cooked dry legumes   __days
nuts and seeds   __days
plain fermented dairy products   __days
I walked   __min/mi   __days
  swam   __min/yd   __days
  rowed   __min   __days
  jogged   __min/mi   __days
  did aerobics   __min   __days
  _____   _____   __days

Week #__ Date:_____
I had
fresh or cooked vegetables   __days
fresh fruits   __days
100 % whole grain   __days
cooked dry legumes   __days
nuts and seeds   __days
plain fermented dairy products   __days
I walked   __min/mi   __days
  swam   __min/yd   __days
  rowed   __min   __days
  jogged   __min/mi   __days
  did aerobics   __min   __days
  _____   _____   __days

Week #__ Date:_____
I had
fresh or cooked vegetables   __days
fresh fruits   __days
100 % whole grain   __days
cooked dry legumes   __days
nuts and seeds   __days
plain fermented dairy products   __days
I walked   __min/mi   __days
  swam   __min/yd   __days
  rowed   __min   __days
  jogged   __min/mi   __days
  did aerobics   __min   __days
  _____   _____   __days

Week #__ Date:_____
I had
fresh or cooked vegetables   __days
fresh fruits   __days
100 % whole grain   __days
cooked dry legumes   __days
nuts and seeds   __days
plain fermented dairy products   __days
I walked   __min/mi   __days
  swam   __min/yd   __days
  rowed   __min   __days
  jogged   __min/mi   __days
  did aerobics   __min   __days
  _____   _____   __days

Week #__ Date:_____
I had
fresh or cooked vegetables   __days
fresh fruits   __days
100 % whole grain   __days
cooked dry legumes   __days
nuts and seeds   __days
plain fermented dairy products   __days
I walked   __min/mi   __days
  swam   __min/yd   __days
  rowed   __min   __days
  jogged   __min/mi   __days
  did aerobics   __min   __days
  _____   _____   __days

Week #__ Date:_____
I had
fresh or cooked vegetables   __days
fresh fruits   __days
100 % whole grain   __days
cooked dry legumes   __days
nuts and seeds   __days
plain fermented dairy products   __days
I walked   __min/mi   __days
  swam   __min/yd   __days
  rowed   __min   __days
  jogged   __min/mi   __days
  did aerobics   __min   __days
  _____   _____   __days

Week #__ Date:_____
I had
fresh or cooked vegetables   __days
fresh fruits   __days
100 % whole grain   __days
cooked dry legumes   __days
nuts and seeds   __days
plain fermented dairy products   __days
I walked   __min/mi   __days
  swam   __min/yd   __days
  rowed   __min   __days
  jogged   __min/mi   __days
  did aerobics   __min   __days
  _____   _____   __days

Week #__ Date:_____
I had
fresh or cooked vegetables   __days
fresh fruits   __days
100 % whole grain   __days
cooked dry legumes   __days
nuts and seeds   __days
plain fermented dairy products   __days
I walked   __min/mi   __days
  swam   __min/yd   __days
  rowed   __min   __days
  jogged   __min/mi   __days
  did aerobics   __min   __days
  _____   _____   __days

Week #__ Date:_____
I had
fresh or cooked vegetables   __days
fresh fruits   __days
100 % whole grain   __days
cooked dry legumes   __days
nuts and seeds   __days
plain fermented dairy products   __days
I walked   __min/mi   __days
   swam   __min/yd   __days
   rowed   __min   __days
   jogged   __min/mi   __days
   did aerobics   __min   __days
   _____   _____   __days

Week #__ Date:_____
I had
fresh or cooked vegetables   __days
fresh fruits   __days
100 % whole grain   __days
cooked dry legumes   __days
nuts and seeds   __days
plain fermented dairy products   __days
I walked   __min/mi   __days
   swam   __min/yd   __days
   rowed   __min   __days
   jogged   __min/mi   __days
   did aerobics   __min   __days
   _____   _____   __days

Week #__ Date:_____
I had
fresh or cooked vegetables   __days
fresh fruits   __days
100 % whole grain   __days
cooked dry legumes   __days
nuts and seeds   __days
plain fermented dairy products   __days
I walked   __min/mi   __days
    swam   __min/yd   __days
    rowed   __min   __days
    jogged   __min/mi   __days
    did aerobics   __min   __days
    _____   _____   __days

Week #__ Date:_____
I had
fresh or cooked vegetables   __days
fresh fruits   __days
100 % whole grain   __days
cooked dry legumes   __days
nuts and seeds   __days
plain fermented dairy products   __days
I walked   __min/mi   __days
    swam   __min/yd   __days
    rowed   __min   __days
    jogged   __min/mi   __days
    did aerobics   __min   __days
    _____   _____   __days

BIBLIOGRAPHY

Airola, Paavo: *Hypoglycemia: a better approach* - Phoenix, Health Plus Publishers, 1986

Benet, Sula: *How to live to be 100 - The life-style of the people of the Caucasus* - New York, The Dial Press, 1976

Brody, Jane: *Jane Brody's Good Food Book* - New York, W.W. Norton & Co., 1985

Buchman, Dian Dincin: *Herbal medicine* - Philadelphia, George F. Stickley & Co., 1981

Dadd, Debra Lynn: *The nontoxic home* - Los Angeles, Jeremy P. Tarcher, Inc., 1986

Dadd, Debra Lynn: *Nontoxic and Natural* - Los Angeles, Jeremy P. Tarcher, Inc., 1984

Diet, Nutrition, and Cancer - Washington D.C., National Academy Press, 1982

Encyclopedia of food additives - Globe Communications Corp., 1987

Family Cookbook, Volume II. - Englewood Cliffs, Prentice-Hall, Inc., 1984

Farquhar, John W.: *The American way of life need not be hazardous to your health* - New York, W.W. Norton & Co., 1978

Halsell, Grace: *Los Viejos: Secrets of long life from the Sacred Valley* - Emmaus, Rodale Press, Inc., 1976

McQeen-Williams, Morvyth and Apisson, Barbara: *A diet for 100 healthy happy years* - Englewood Cliffs, Prentice-Hall, Inc., 1977

Ness, Joanne: *The Calcium-requirement cookbook* - M. Evans and Company, Inc. New York, 1985

The People's Guide to Vitamins and Minerals - Contemporary Books, Inc. Chicago, 1980

Reuben, David: *Everything you always wanted to know about nutrition* - New York, Avon Publishers, 1979

Reuben, David: *The save your life diet* - New York, Random House, 1975

Stern, Judith S. and Denenberg, R.V.: *How to stay slim and healthy on the fast food diet* - Englewood Cliffs, Prentice-Hall, Inc., 1980

Uvezian, Sonia: *The book of Yogurt* - San Francisco, 101 Productions, 1978

Uvezian, Sonia: *Cooking from the Caucasus* - New York, Harcourt Brace Jovanovich, Inc., 1978

NOTES

NOTES

NOTES